Principles of Evolutionary Medicine

Principles of Evolutionary Medicine

Peter Gluckman

Centre for Human Evolution, Adaptation and Disease, Liggins Institute,
The University of Auckland, New Zealand

Alan Beedle

Centre for Human Evolution, Adaptation and Disease, Liggins Institute,
The University of Auckland, New Zealand

Mark Hanson

Institute of Developmental Sciences, University of Southampton, UK

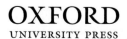

OXFORD
UNIVERSITY PRESS

OXFORD
UNIVERSITY PRESS

Great Clarendon Street, Oxford OX2 6DP

Oxford University Press is a department of the University of Oxford.
It furthers the University's objective of excellence in research, scholarship,
and education by publishing worldwide in

Oxford New York

Auckland Cape Town Dar es Salaam Hong Kong Karachi
Kuala Lumpur Madrid Melbourne Mexico City Nairobi
New Delhi Shanghai Taipei Toronto

With offices in

Argentina Austria Brazil Chile Czech Republic France Greece
Guatemala Hungary Italy Japan Poland Portugal Singapore
South Korea Switzerland Thailand Turkey Ukraine Vietnam

Oxford is a registered trade mark of Oxford University Press
in the UK and in certain other countries

Published in the United States
by Oxford University Press Inc., New York

British Library Cataloguing in Publication Data

Data available

Library of Congress Cataloging in Publication Data

Data available

Typeset by Newgen Imaging Systems (P) Ltd., Chennai, India
Printed in Great Britain
on acid-free paper by
CPI Antony Rowe, Chippenham, Wiltshire

ISBN 978-0-19-923638-1(Hbk.)
      978-0-19-923639-8(Pbk.)

10 9 8 7 6 5 4 3 2

Contents

promote passage of genetic information from one generation to the next and evolutionary success is about successful passage of genes within a lineage to future generations. Thus the processes of evolution are focused on what drives reproductive success within a lineage, a concept termed fitness. But fitness does not depend necessarily on longevity or health. It involves trade-offs which ensure reproductive success even if they incur other costs such as a shorter life. Evolutionary biology is a science that considers how an organism trades-off one component of its biology against others to optimize its fitness. Because many modern humans live long lives and medicine is increasingly focused on promoting the quality of life, health professionals cannot ignore the constraints imposed by such evolutionary considerations.

Evolutionary medicine, therefore, is a growing and central discipline that applies evolutionary knowledge to the understanding of human biology, both normal and abnormal. It is an essential science, necessary for a holistic perception of how health and disease emerge. It has application in both individual health care and in public health. It adds much to understanding other basic disciplines of medicine, including physiology, anatomy, biochemistry, pathology, molecular biology, population health, and behavioural sciences. Indeed, a complete understanding of these more immediate disciplines is not possible without an understanding of evolutionary biology.

Evolutionary biology is a vibrant, if broad, domain of biomedical science. Some aspects of evolutionary knowledge are not essential or central to understanding the core principles of evolutionary medicine. For example, the subject of macroevolution – the process underpinning speciation and biodiversity – is not central to a medical perspective. Much of evolutionary biology involves quantitative approaches, for example for defining aspects of selection or genetic drift; again, these are not essential for the medical reader. Many of the details of the dynamics of selective processes are technical and are not required in applying evolutionary principles in human medicine. We have therefore omitted them from this book, which is intended for the clinician, whether in training or in practice. Most textbooks in evolutionary biology focus on other species and only minimally refer to the human. In contrast, unless there is an essential comparative point to be made, we have tried to use only examples from human biology to illustrate key evolutionary principles.

The book is presented in three parts. In the first we detail the basic principles of evolutionary biology: what biological evolution is, how it operates through the processes of selection, how evolution is reflected in our genome, the relationship between genotype and phenotype, how developmental and evolutionary processes interact, what determines the characteristics of the human life history, and how the evolution of our species has led to features which now become manifest in the doctor's office or on the hospital ward. An important evolved characteristic of our species is that we live in groups and our social environment and our capacity to develop and apply technology are essential components of our evolution. So it is not possible to discuss biological evolution without consideration of our cultural evolution and this we do in the first part of the book.

In the second part of the book we describe how these principles can be applied to an understanding of human disease, using four illustrative axes: human reproduction; nutrition and metabolism; biological defence systems; and human behaviour. We have intentionally restricted the discussion in this way so that these systems can be elucidated in sufficient detail to highlight how evolutionary approaches to the human condition can be applied in practice. This is not intended to be a comprehensive medical textbook – there are plenty of those – but is intended to give the reader a new understanding which can be applied generally in clinical medicine and which informs other domains of medical science.

In the third part of the book, we synthesize these various strands to provide a systematic evolutionary framework for understanding human health and disease. We propose that each person presenting to a physician has three relevant histories: the history of the complaint itself; the developmental history of that individual; and his or her evolutionary history. All three histories are essential for a comprehensive understanding of the way an individual has responded to his or her environment. We detail the pathways by which individual risk can be influenced by evolutionary processes, pathways which should always be part of a health professional's reflection on the situation of the patient before him/her.

Evolutionary biology has an intimate relationship with the ecological sciences and humans must also be understood in their ecological context. Consideration of how our lives progress in any environment, including our social environment, is greatly enhanced by understanding evolutionary biology. In turn, such understanding can contribute greatly to the development of effective public health strategies.

Evolutionary biology as a science has always had, and continues to have, an awkward and complex relationship with broader intellectual and philosophical concerns. For example, it is seen by some to be in conflict with their specific belief systems. Darwin's propositions when first put forward were clearly at odds with the prevailing concepts of natural theology and of an active creation, the dominant institutional explanations of the natural world in early nineteenth century Britain. Yet today the majority of scientists find no need to see evolutionary biology as in conflict with their personal beliefs, and most religious authorities find no conflict between their theology and the science of evolution. Like modern astronomy, evolutionary science is a robust and mature science and, without it, human biology cannot be fully appreciated. The biology and the conceptual frameworks of evolutionary science are incontrovertible, but what they *mean* to individuals or particular faith groups is a quite distinct and in many ways unrelated issue. Many patients and indeed many doctors have a devout faith and this book does not set out to challenge that faith. Rather, it wishes to impart to those who have a responsibility for medical care and public health the principles of a biological science which is necessary for integrating the other basic and applied medical sciences. Without it, medicine cannot progress, any more than it could until the inaccurate anatomical teaching of Galen in the second century had been superseded.

Evolutionary concepts have been wrongly and inappropriately applied beyond biology, particularly in political contexts. In these circumstances a metaphorical understanding (or more often a misunderstanding) of evolutionary science has been applied in an inappropriate context. Anarchists on one hand and fascists on the other co-opted evolutionary thought to their political ideology. Because such abuses still occur today, health professionals will encounter them. In the final chapter of this book we will briefly discuss these issues.

Each of the authors has a long history of research in aspects of evolutionary biology and medicine. But none of us is an expert in all its aspects: it is a large field. We are grateful to the many colleagues who directly or indirectly have contributed to our understanding and thus to this volume. One person in particular, Dr Chris Kuzawa (Northwestern University, Chicago, IL, USA), was critical to the book. Chris made major contributions to Chapters 5 and 8 in the early stages. Unfortunately other commitments prevented him from playing the larger role which we, and he, had planned. We must also acknowledge colleagues who have read chapters, offered critiques and suggestions, and elucidated matters beyond our expertise. They include Professor Sir Patrick Bateson FRS (Cambridge), Professor Peter Ellison (Harvard), Professor Eva Jablonka (Tel Aviv), Professor Hamish Spencer (Dunedin), Professor Randolph Nesse (Michigan), Professor Paul Rainey (Massey), Professor Russell Gray (Auckland), Professor Wayne Cutfield (Auckland), Professor Murray Mitchell (Auckland), and Professor Des Gorman (Auckland). We thank Dr Cinda Cupido (Auckland), Dr Tatjana Buklijas (Auckland), Dr Felicia Low (Auckland), and Ms Amanda Calhoun (Yale) for assistance with research.

Peter Gluckman
Alan Beedle
Mark Hanson
October 2008

Part 1

Fundamentals of evolutionary biology

CHAPTER 1

Introduction

Life expectancy in developed societies has risen dramatically over the past 250 years as a result of major technological changes, including improvements in public health and in the understanding of the biology of disease, and through concurrent societal changes which have brought a greater emphasis on the value of life. Life expectancy at birth in pre-revolutionary France was about 30 years – not so different from that of prehistoric (and in particular Palaeolithic; see Table 1.1) humans – yet now it is about 80 years. Advances in nutrition, infection control and treatment, trauma care, and maternity and neonatal services have addressed many of the extrinsic causes of death that led to the short lifespan of our Palaeolithic forebears. These causes also largely contributed to what we now call 'premature' death in our not-so-distant ancestors (Figure 1.1). But as we live longer, diseases which were previously unimportant become more so; many of them, such as cardiovascular disease, appearing in middle age, at an age when the majority of our forebears were already dead. Other morbidities such as mental disorders have become more dominant as a result of the pressures of living in the much more complex societal structure that urbanization has brought.

In addition, our ambitions as organisms have changed: advances in medical care, improved access to knowledge, and individual empowerment have brought a focus on longevity and quality of life. Modern medicine is increasingly faced with the patient's expectation of being able to live well into their ninth decade and to expect highly interventional medicine if needed to maintain quality of life throughout. Increasingly we face causes of disability which do not arise from extrinsic causes of disease but result from intrinsic ageing of cellular processes, as reflected in degenerative disease. Thus, while medicine is now dominated by a population-wide expectation of good health into old age, this to a large extent is in conflict with the evolutionary processes that moulded our species. This textbook is about the principles underlying those processes and how many disease states can be understood in terms of this conflict. While health and longevity are the primary concern of our patients, neither of these, with caveats to be discussed later, are the primary drivers of evolutionary processes.

Briefly stated, evolution of a species (**macroevolution**) and evolutionary change within a species (**microevolution**) operate to produce an organism that is matched or adapted to its environment; that match is not defined by a particularly long or comfortable life for an individual, but rather on the successful passage of that individual's genes to successive generations. Indeed it is a truism that all organisms on the planet today are here because their ancestors reproduced successfully. Lineages that did not do so are now extinct. This is the core concept of **fitness**, which is fundamental to evolutionary biology. Evolution is the process whereby a population changes over time to optimize fitness of its individual members within a particular environment, so *Homo sapiens* largely evolved by adaptations that maximized its fitness in the environments of eastern Africa, the region in which our species first emerged. Biological fitness for a human was – and still is – achieved by a strategy of supporting a small number of progeny to grow successfully to adulthood, reproduce and live long enough to support their own offspring becoming reproductively competent. Evolutionary pressures on our lineage operated to ensure this: there were few if any drivers of health beyond the

Table 1.1 Approximate human and geological timescales expressed in thousands of years before present (KYA). Definitions for human timescales can vary depending on region.

Human timescale			Geological epoch
Period		KYA	
Palaeolithic	Lower	2500–100/200	Pliocene (5300–1800 KYA) and Pleistocene (1800–10 KYA)
	Middle	300–30	
	Upper	50–10	
Mesolithic		10–6	Holocene (10 KYA–present)
Neolithic		10–4	
Bronze age		5.3–2.4	
Iron age		3.3–1.6	

reproductive period in the life course, or generally of longevity beyond the period necessary to support offspring into adulthood.

The term **environment** occurs frequently throughout this book, and a definition here is thus appropriate. Evolutionary and developmental biologists use the term in a wider sense than is common by popular usage, where it relates to issues such as global warming or threatened biodiversity. We define the environment of an organism as the sum of all the external conditions and stimuli that it experiences, including climate, nutrient supply, social structure resulting from cooperation with or competition from other members of its own species, and threats from other species in the form of predation, parasitism, or infection. If the environment changes for the worse, the lineage may be able to cope but at a cost; or it may go extinct; or individuals may adapt to their new environment, or (if mobile) may be able migrate to a more matched environment. Some species can ensure relative constancy of their environment by constructing it themselves, a process called **niche construction**; for example, the temperature-controlling mounds of termites or the dams constructed by beavers. The human species is a niche constructor *par excellence* through its use of technologies ranging from fire and clothing to urban design and, as described in numerous places in this book, this capability has both positive and negative consequences for our health.

1.1 What is disease?

Whereas modern medicine focuses on concepts of health, evolutionary biology focuses on the determinants

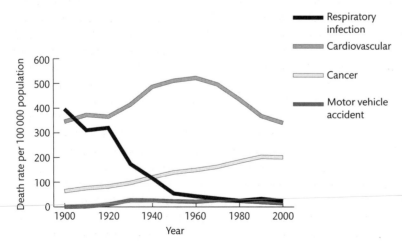

Figure 1.1 Causes of death have changed in the twentieth century in the USA. Data from US Public Health Service, Vital Statistics Reports.

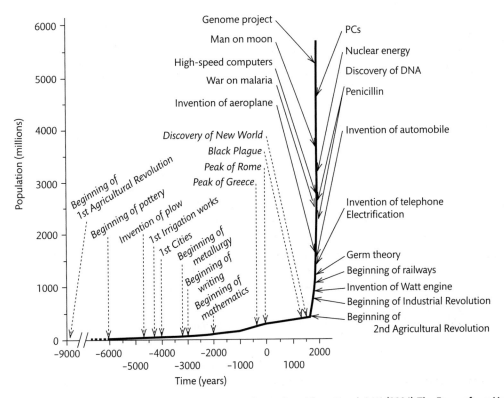

Figure 1.3 Anthropogenic changes in the human environment (reproduced from Fogel, R.W. (2004) *The Escape from Hunger and Premature Death, 1700–2100: Europe, America and the Third World.* Cambridge University Press, with permission).

can encourage such thinking. To do so is a form of **teleology**. There is a major difference in the thought processes underlying the statement that 'limbs evolved for walking', which is teleological, and the evolutionary statement that 'there was progressive selection over time on the traits associated with the ancestral fin, and the adaptive advantage associated with effective terrestrial movement led to cumulative selective change resulting in the formation of the limb'. But we can see how clumsy the second statement is, so it is easy to be sloppy and say that a process or a structure 'evolved for…'. It is an almost unavoidable temptation, but when we do so we must also remember that this does not imply purpose.

The beginning of modern evolutionary theory in the late eighteenth century was the growing acceptance of two fundamental concepts. The first was gradualism, the idea that the geological features of the planet are the result of slow processes operating over 'deep time'. The second was that biological species are not immutable but that, with time, new species could emerge, could evolve into other species, or could become extinct, and that, in biology as well as geology, deep time provides a setting for such gradual change. Although macroevolution is a large component of evolutionary biology, it is not a major focus of this book beyond a brief consideration of the evolutionary history of the hominoid lineage since the last common ancestor of *Homo* and chimpanzees (Chapter 6). But Charles Darwin recognized that species could change their characteristics over time, and we term this within-species change **microevolution**. Importantly, macroevolution and microevolution are a continuum, not distinct processes. Classically, evolution is therefore defined as 'change with time within a population of organisms over generations', and the insights of Charles Darwin and his correspondent and competitor Alfred Russell Wallace were to see that this change is a result of **selection** acting on heritable variation in the **traits** of a population.

Most evolutionary biology has focused on genetic inheritance. Indeed, it was the discovery of the gene as providing a mechanism for inheritance which eventually moved selection to the centre of biological thinking. However, as we will discuss later in the book, there are other modes of inheritance, and increasingly these have been incorporated into evolutionary science.

1.2.1 Selection

Selection describes the processes by which one individual is more likely to reproduce successfully than another within a population because of the presence of a particular advantageous trait. It is itself a word which has metaphorical danger. If there is a genetically inherited component to that particular trait, then that particular trait will become concentrated in the next generation of that population. Darwin's seminal contribution was to recognize the importance of selection. He introduced his most famous book, *On the Origin of Species by Means of Natural Selection, or the Preservation of Favoured Races in the Struggle for Life* (shortened in later editions to *The Origin of Species*), with a discussion of **artificial selection**, which is the form of selection known to plant or animal breeders who select for a particularly desirable trait by breeding from individuals with a variation in that trait in the desired direction. Artificial selection, as with the other forms of selection, can only operate to the extent that it is heritable, and it was Darwin's observations of animal breeding which gave him insights into this process, even though there was as yet no widely accepted theory of how inheritance might operate (Darwin did not know of the work of Gregor Mendel: see below and Chapter 2). In *The Origin of Species* Darwin makes one of the greatest intellectual leaps in science to recognize that selective processes also operate in nature. He recognized that natural variation in a trait might make an individual organism more or less likely to survive and reproduce successfully in a given environment and that therefore as that trait became concentrated in the population over time the lineage would evolve to be well adapted to a particular environment. He called this process **natural selection** by analogy with artificial selection. But whereas artificial selection has a direction determined by the selective agent (the breeder), any direction in natural selection is solely determined by the selecting environment.

Darwin recognized that selection is about reproductive success. Natural selection is one mechanism to achieve this, but in his second major book, *The Descent of Man, and Selection in Relation to Sex*, Darwin described a second mechanism, whereby reproductive success is not related to characteristics affecting survival but rather to sexual dominance and choice. In a species where there is competition (usually among males) for mating opportunity, individuals may fight for sexual dominance and thus there is **sexual selection** for body size and strength. For example, the male elephant seal is much larger than the female. In other species, particularly birds, mating choice by the female may be dependent on the physical appearance of the male and this can lead to the evolution of sexually dimorphic extravagances such as the peacock's tail. We will discuss sexual selection in relationship to human biology in several later chapters.

1.2.2 Variation and inheritance

The key features of the above discussion are the themes of variation and inheritance. Recognition of their importance was another of Darwin's seminal contributions. Up to his time, biologists (and doctors) had largely been concerned with *classifying* all living organisms and they therefore concentrated on similarities – as defining the average for a species – rather than variations. Darwin shifted the focus to individual variation *within* a species. The most remarkable aspect of the contributions of Darwin and the other early evolutionists including Wallace is that they made their observations in the absence of any understanding of how variation and inheritance might operate.

It was the discovery of particulate inheritance – the idea that characteristics could be inherited as discrete units – that led to the development of genetics and the study of mutation. The field was slow to develop because the principles of inheritance elucidated by Gregor Mendel were ignored for 20 years until they were rediscovered at the beginning of the twentieth century. There were bitter disagreements between selectionist biologists and genetic biologists until the Modern Synthesis (see Chapter 2) brought these two fields together into an integrated concept. The discovery of DNA and the power of molecular biology added impetus to this integration. In particular these

---

Box 1.3   Seeking similarities or seeking differences

Humans have long classified living things on the basis of their appearance, behaviour or habitat, but our present understanding of biological species owes much to the work of two scientists whose lives were separated by just 100 years, the eighteenth-century Swedish naturalist Carl Linnaeus (1707–1778) and the nineteenth-century English naturalist Charles Darwin (1809–1882).

In 1758, Linnaeus published his *Systema Naturae*, a book describing all the then known species of plants and animals and also containing a scheme for classifying them: the Linnaean System of taxonomy with its hierarchy of species, genera, families, orders, classes, phyla and kingdoms. Linnaeus introduced the binomial system of species names – for example *Homo sapiens* – and proposed that species are the fundamental unit of classification. Although he recognized that species are usually classified by morphology – members of a species tend to resemble each other more than they resemble members of other species – he appreciated that the underlying definition of a species is the ability of individuals within a species to interbreed and produce viable offspring. Linnaeus's

world view was that species were fixed and immutable, and that each species had been created by a higher power to fill a place in the sequential ladder of life.

Any biography of Charles Darwin will recount the story of how his desire to be viewed as a credible biologist consisted of a 7-year study of the taxonomy of barnacles. That endeavour taught Darwin that within a given species there is a wide spectrum of variation, and that it is often difficult to decide where variation within a species shades into a distinct species. The appreciation of such variation helped to reinforce his developing view that species were not immutable and that selective retention of beneficial variation might be a mechanism for one species to change into another.

The Linnean Society of London, the world's oldest learned society devoted solely to natural history, takes its name from Linnaeus and maintains his botanical, zoological, and library collections. The papers by Darwin and Wallace first proposing the theory of evolution by means of natural selection were read at a meeting of the Linnean Society on 1 July 1858.

---

discoveries provided a mechanism for heritable variation, but molecular architecture also provides powerful evidence for how evolution has progressed. When used in relation to speciation, for example, the evidence from DNA goes far beyond the fossil records with which Darwin and his colleagues had to content themselves. In Chapters 3 and 6 we review how we can use our understanding of the gene both to explain and demonstrate evolution and to explore evolutionary history. Subsequent evolutionary research has essentially built on these fundamental principles to describe the origin of variation: to what extent it is driven by mutation, the link between genotype and phenotype, the role of chance, the speed of evolution, the level at which selection operates, and the modes of inheritance.

1.2.3 Development and the life course

However, one area of biology was more difficult to include in the synthesis between molecular and selectionist thinking, and that is the impact of developmental processes, operating from conception to maturity. Development is not simply a matter of a fertilized ovum growing and dividing according to a pre-programmed mechanism. There are complex pathways of differentiation from a single cell into an adult human and there are distinct components to the life course: from pre-implantation embryo, to implanted embryo, to fetus, to neonate, to dependent infant, to juvenile, adolescent, and adult. In recent years, major progress has been made in integrating our understanding of **developmental plasticity** – a set of processes which have themselves evolved – with the remainder of evolutionary thought.

Organisms have different biological strategies at different times in their lives. Some organisms have very distinct forms and can have very complex life courses: for example, the human parasites causing malaria (a protozoan) and schistosomiasis (a flatworm) have multiple forms according to whether they are living in humans or in their invertebrate vectors (mosquitoes and water snails, respectively). Humans too have distinct phases in their life courses. For example, the nutritional processes of the pre-implantation embryo, fetus, pre-weaning infant, and adult are all very different. The human fetus is nourished across the placenta so both placental physiology and the mother's adaptations to pregnancy are attuned to maximize the nutrition of the fetus. The fetal gastrointestinal tract is quiescent until birth, at which time it is activated and uniquely adapted for digestion of human milk, for example of lactose using lactase. After weaning, human gastrointestinal physiology changes yet again, one feature being the bulk of the world's population losing lactase activity.

One component of evolutionary biology is to consider how different phases in the life course evolved and how these different phases are inter-related. An organism's life-course strategy is ultimately an issue of using energy supplies optimally to maximize reproductive success, so selection operates on components of this balance, such as investment in growth, pattern of development, approach to reproduction, social structure, and pattern of ageing, all aimed at maximizing fitness within the environment of the population. **Trade-offs** must be made, given the limiting availability of energy and the constraints of time: the risk of death from predation or disease before reproduction. Body size itself is constrained by mechanical, nutrient-availability, or thermoregulatory issues. The section of evolutionary biology related to consideration of these general strategies and trade-offs is known as **life history theory**. Humans have very distinct characteristics to their life history traits, and these and their medical implications are discussed in Chapter 5.

Just as selection is the process of the interaction between inherited determinants of phenotype and the

---

Box 1.4 Parasitic life cycles

Many parasites have complex life cycles, which can involve both free-living phases as well as parasitic phases in one of several different hosts. Why and how would parasites evolve to such complexity? The advantages of multiple or intermediate hosts may include resistance to extinction of one host species as well as improved dispersal or transmission. Complex life cycles are likely to evolve by capturing a new host, which requires the existing and new hosts to be sharing an environment. For example, it may be that the concentration of humans into settlements during the Neolithic (agricultural) revolution about 11 000 years ago created a shared environment for humans and mosquitoes that allowed the malaria parasite to become a major human pathogen.

The malaria parasite, various species of the protozoan *Plasmodium*, uses humans as host and the *Anopheles* mosquito as an intermediate vector.

The life cycle begins when an infected mosquito bites a human. Sporozoite forms of the parasite from the mosquito salivary gland are injected into the human along with the mosquito's anticoagulant saliva. The sporozoites move through the bloodstream to the liver and penetrate and multiply within hepatocytes, where they remain for several days. Next they return to the blood and penetrate red blood cells, in which they produce either merozoites, which can reinfect the liver and red blood cells, or the reproductive form of the parasite, gametocytes. If another mosquito feeds on the infected human, the gametocytes in the ingested blood self-fertilize in the insect's gut and an oocyst develops in the gut wall. The oocyst ruptures to produce many sporozoites, which migrate to the mosquito's salivary gland to complete the cycle.

environment, development is not a solely intrinsic process in which a single ovum grows into a mature organism. Rather the developing organism is subject to external influences which affect its later phenotype (see Chapter 4). Vulnerability to such influences is enhanced during particular critical windows of development, which occur at different stages according to the nature of the environmental stimulus. At the most pathological level, exposure of the developing embryo to certain drugs can interfere with cell replication and interaction. For example, the anticancer drug methotrexate, which crosses the placenta and interferes with folic acid metabolism, can cause spontaneous abortion (at high doses) and fetal defects (at moderate to low doses), particularly when given shortly before conception or in the first trimester of pregnancy. This is a pathological example, but environmental variation within the normal range can also affect fetal development. For example, severe famine during pregnancy can lead to children who are born small, and as we will see in Chapter 8 this has consequences for their health throughout their lives.

1.3   Time

Organisms face challenges over a number of timescales. These include immediate physical challenges, such as intraspecific competition for energy and reproductive opportunity or attack by predators (themselves engaged in energy harvesting), and changes in the environment. The latter may be short-term, such as daily temperature fluctuations, medium-term such as seasonality of food availability, or long-term such as climate change causing disappearance of preferred food sources or habitat.

Organisms have evolved a hierarchy of responses to these challenges. Some classical homeostatic responses are very rapid and highly reversible (e.g. those mediated by the central nervous and endocrine systems) over seconds to hours, and some involve structural change or long-term readjustment of set points for homeostatic feedback systems (called rheostasis) and these operate over hours to years. Many of these longer-term but within-lifetime effects are initiated in early life through the processes of developmental plasticity. Yet other responses are beyond the timescale of individual lifetimes and involve natural selection, resulting in genetic change (Figure 1.4) over several generations.

An example of a short-term (homeostatic) response is sweating or shivering in response to temperature change. Increased muscle size, perfusion with blood, and changes in myofibre metabolism after physical training provide an example of a medium-term and reversible plastic response affecting tissue function or organization. The development of active sweat glands represents an example of developmental plasticity: sweat glands are innervated in the first few weeks after birth and the density of innervation and thus the capacity to sweat and tolerate extreme heat is influenced by whether the infant is brought up in a warm or cold environment. The consequences are a different capacity to tolerate heat stress as adults. Humans from lineages that stayed in tropical Africa from our initial appearance as a species have generally different body shapes to those from lineages that have lived in higher-latitude environments for many millennia. Here selective pressures are likely to have favoured different body shapes to aid thermoregulation in the very different climates these lineages have faced (see Chapter 6).

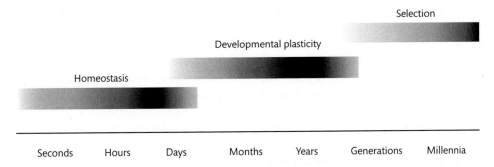

Figure 1.4 Responses over different timescales (reproduced from Gluckman *et al., Lancet* 2009, in press, with permission).

As another example of temporally different classes of response, consider the hierarchy of responses affecting that most extensive and sensitive of human organs: the skin. We respond to a pinprick with immediate withdrawal, on a timescale of less than a second, mediated by cutaneous nociceptors. On a slightly longer timescale of minutes to hours, another insult – ultraviolet radiation – causes sunburn characterized by erythema, pain, and oedema. That also invokes a behavioural avoidance response: we cover our skin. The sensitivity of skin to ultraviolet radiation is determined by its content of melanin, and for many people with light skin the melanin content can be increased by a medium-term adaptive response that increases output from melanocytes, so a suntan develops over days to weeks. And long-term genetic adaptations of human populations to the amounts of sunlight at different latitudes have created a variety of human skin colours caused by variation in the amount and type of melanin in the skin. It is likely that the selective pressure for lighter skin colour in populations living at higher latitudes arose from the need to preserve vitamin D synthesis in the skin in areas of lower sunlight availability. But this can result in vitamin D deficiency in darker-skinned migrant populations, especially when traditional concealing clothing is worn by women.

It is also important to appreciate how responses on the shorter timescales can be modified by an individual's previous developmental experience or evolutionary

---

Box 1.5 Vitamin D and skin pigmentation

Vitamin D is critical to bone formation and deficiency causes rickets in children and osteomalacia in adults. Vitamin D is synthesized in the skin after exposure to ultraviolet irradiation, or can be obtained from the diet. Any factor that reduces exposure to photons in the ultraviolet frequency range, such as skin pigmentation, use of sunscreens, or concealing clothing, will reduce vitamin D synthesis and may lead to deficiency. The geographic distribution of skin pigmentation in humans is primarily determined by exposure to ultraviolet radiation, with an almost linear relationship between latitude of population origin and skin reflectance. Explanations for this clinal gradient generally invoke natural selection favouring high pigmentation, and therefore protection from ultraviolet-induced skin damage, in areas of high sun exposure and conversely decreased pigmentation, and therefore increased vitamin D synthesis, in areas of low sun exposure.

In high-latitude regions (including the UK and large parts of North America), there is insufficient ultraviolet radiation during a substantial part of the year to allow vitamin D synthesis, even for light-skinned people. Consequently, there is a high prevalence of vitamin D insufficiency (serum levels of 25-hydroxyvitamin D less than 40–50 nmol/L) in people in these areas. People with dark skin require up to 10 times more exposure to sunlight than those with light skin to produce the same amount of vitamin D, and consequently the prevalence of insufficiency is higher in those populations. For example, prevalence rates of 52–76% for African-Americans, 18–50% in Hispanics, and 8–31% in Europids were recently recorded in a US study. Surprisingly, vitamin D levels have been found to be positively associated with latitude in Europe, with highest levels in Scandinavian countries and lowest levels in Southern Europe; this may be a result of cultural (sun exposure seeking versus avoidance), socio-economic (use of vitamin supplements), and dietary (high consumption of fish, which is an excellent dietary source of vitamin D) factors.

Even in sunny countries such as Australia and parts of the Middle East, the prevalence of vitamin D insufficiency may be as high as 80% among dark-skinned women who clothe their bodies entirely for cultural reasons. Such trends may be associated with the re-emergence of rickets in such communities. These results are leading to calls for reconsideration of guidelines for sun exposure and for vitamin D supplementation.

history. For example, susceptibility to sunburn is modified by past exposure (suntan) and by population origin (skin colour). Susceptibility to the effects of milk consumption is modified by developmental stage (lactase is lost during development) and by ancestral nutritional history. These examples underline the importance of a complete knowledge of an individual's history for understanding their current health status.

1.4   Constraints

Evolution is not without limits. Such **constraints** may arise from the nature of physical processes. For example, insects are – perhaps fortunately for human survival on the planet – limited in size by gravity, the mechanics of their exoskeleton, and the physics of oxygen diffusion along their tracheal network. Or constraints can arise because evolution generally works in an incremental way: for example, the human eye is poorly 'designed', but gradual evolution towards the structure of the superficially similar but optically superior octopus eye would require non-functioning intermediate forms, so we have retained the organizational structure of our eye in a form modified from functioning eyes in our precursor lineage. In addition we must remember that most of the discussion so far has been about qualitative aspects of the environment. But constraints will also act when there is a mismatch between the *rate* of environmental change and that at which natural selection can operate, or simply from an extreme *degree* of environmental change.

The complexity of the link between the **genotype** and **phenotype** places all sorts of constraints on how selection can operate. As will be reviewed in Chapter 3, the concept of a single gene relating to a single trait is in general misleading. Single-gene effects may lead to mutations and disease, but selection operates on the integrated phenotype and this creates limitations on the rate and nature of change between generations. Consider human childbirth. As discussed in detail in Chapter 7, the human pelvis has quite a distinct shape compared to that of other apes. This is because we are bipedal and the mechanics of efficient walking and running have led to selection of relatively rotated hips and a narrower pelvis. Yet there has to be a trade-off, because humans are also distinguished by a large brain. Thus if birth occurred

---

Box 1.6   What is a clade?

A clade is defined as a cluster of species that all descended from a common precursor species. The field of **cladistics** groups organisms hierarchically according to evolutionary relationships. Genomic analysis has replaced morphological analysis in cladistic analysis. The goal of cladistic analysis is to identify how species diverged from common ancestors and where novel features appeared or others were lost. The last common ancestor of humans and the other great apes existed about 15 million years ago. Cladistic analysis shows that the orangutan first diverged in its evolution, followed by the gorilla, followed by the two species of chimpanzee (Figure 1.5).

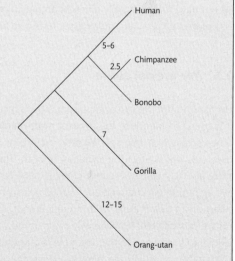

Figure 1.5 The hominoid clade, showing calculated dates of divergence in millions of years.

at the same stage of neuronal maturation as in other apes, with well-developed motor function at birth, the head would be too large to pass through the pelvic outlet. Hence, while other apes are **precocial** (that is, have relatively mature offspring at birth capable of a level of independent activity), humans have developed secondary **altricial** characteristics and are extremely dependent on the mother for a long period after birth. Here is an example where a constraint was imposed on how human evolution could proceed by the development of bipedalism early in the evolution of the hominin clade (see Chapter 6).

There are also constraints imposed by biochemical and physiological processes which have in turn been imposed by the past evolution of that lineage. For example, human physiology has evolved such that we cannot live and reproduce successfully above about 5000 m and cannot survive at all without supplementary oxygen above 9000 m. In contrast, the bar-headed goose migrates regularly over the Himalayas at altitudes of up to 10 000 m.

Constraints and **exaptations (**features that perform a function but were not initially selected for their current use; for example, the three small bones of the middle ear originally evolved in jaw-boned fish as part of their jaw hinge mechanism), and 'historical contingencies' (chance events that have determined, for example, why terrestrial life is based on L- rather than D-amino acids and why the human and cephalopod eyes look superficially similar but have fundamentally different architectures), have also played a role in determining our form and function.

1.5 We are not alone

Humans do not live in isolation from other species. Here it is useful to introduce the concept of **co-evolution**, a process by which two species exert reciprocal selective pressures which affect the evolution of both. The lactase story above shows how some humans have evolved to live alongside the cow, and after 10 000 years of artificial selection for milk or meat yield, modern breeds of *Bos taurus* are very different from the wild cattle domesticated by Neolithic humans. A further example is a predator–prey relationship in which the prey evolves some defensive or escape mechanism, and the predator in turn evolves a means of overcoming the response. In predator–prey

interactions, co-evolution can lead to an evolutionary arms race in which the target species must continually change to maintain its fitness relative to the predator species it is co-evolving with. This is the so-called Red Queen effect, named after the character in the children's book *Through the Looking Glass* by Lewis Carroll who complains of always having to run to stay in the same place.

The biggest group of organisms affecting our biology for good or bad is our associated micro-organisms. Infectious disease was a major cause of mortality until the introduction of mass vaccination programmes and antibiotics, very recently in human evolutionary history, and the threat is still with us: the last few decades have seen the emergence of new viral diseases, such as acquired immune deficiency syndrome (AIDS) and severe acute respiratory syndrome (SARS), as well as the resurgence of bacterial diseases once thought to be conquered, such as tuberculosis, now in a lethal multidrug-resistant form. Humans, in common with other vertebrates, have evolved an adaptive immune system to resist infection with micro-organisms, and our antimicrobial phenotype has recently been extended by the use of biotechnology to develop antibiotics and antimicrobial and antiviral drugs. But our pathogens are also engaged in this arms race too, and can use the advantages of vast population sizes and simple genomes to evolve rapidly mechanisms for evading immune surveillance and to neutralize our antimicrobial drugs. As described in Chapter 9, the eventual outcome of that competition often remains uncertain.

Of course, not all micro-organisms are pathogenic. Some, such as yeasts and lactobacilli, have achieved a certain utility in food and beverage preparation, and others are used as chemical reactors in industrial processes after fierce bouts of artificial selection to increase their yield. Other micro-organisms are engaged in a mutual relationship with humans not dissimilar to that between humans and their domesticated animals. The several hundred species of bacteria that comprise the human gut flora perform useful functions, including digestion of some food components, production of vitamins, protection against pathogenic micro-organisms, and fine-tuning of the immune response, in return for life in a stable and protected environment with a regular supply of nutrients. The consequences for health of perturbations in the composition or activity of the gut flora remain largely unexplored.

Fogel, R.W. (2004) *The Escape from Hunger and Premature Death, 1700–2100: Europe, America and the Third World*. Cambridge University Press, Cambridge.

Gilbert, S.F. (2006) *Developmental Biology*. Sinauer Associates, Sunderland, MA.

Quammen, D. (2007) *The Reluctant Mr. Darwin: an Intimate Portrait of Charles Darwin and the Making of his Theory of Evolution*. WW Norton, New York.

Stearns, S.C. (1992) *The Evolution of Life Histories*. Oxford University Press, Oxford.

Stearns, S.C. and Ebert, D. (2001) Evolution in health and disease: work in progress. *Quarterly Review of Biology* **76**, 417–432.

Tishkoff, S.A., Reed, F.A., Ranciaro, A. *et al.* (2007) Convergent adaptation of human lactase persistence in Africa and Europe. *Nature Genetics* **39**, 31–40.

CHAPTER 2

Evolutionary theory

2.1 Introduction

No area of science has produced such a voluminous popular literature, or one as polarized, as evolutionary biology. Perhaps the best comparisons would be with the debates surrounding Copernicus and Galileo in the sixteenth and seventeenth centuries. Both these scholars challenged and ultimately overturned a belief-based system which placed the Earth at the centre of a religiously defined cosmos. In a similar fashion, evolutionary biology has gradually removed the need, once central to the Western religious tradition, to believe that a deity created humans as a special form of organism or controlled the design and macroevolution of the millions of living species, either extinct or extant, that have inhabited the Earth over the past 4 billion years. This statement need not be interpreted as denying (see below) any compatibility between evolutionary biology and religious belief; but evolutionary biology did give impetus to a changed perception of the deity for many people and accelerated a move towards rationalist thought in others. Given the central place that religious belief holds in the psyche for many people, the conceptual challenges that arise from such fundamental changes in perspective, and thus the emotional reaction that they inspire, are understandable.

Evolutionary biology in its essence provides explanations for two sets of phenomena: first how the plethora of species emerged from a single common ancestral species in a series of descendent and radiating lineages, and secondly how organisms come to be well-matched to face the threats and opportunities in the environments they inhabit. Both of these explanations challenge

the concept of deistic creation of individual species and in particular the 'special creation' of *Homo sapiens*; the second also challenges the idea of intentional design of complex organisms. Evolutionary biology requires no agents external to the interaction between the environment and the organism to explain biological complexity and the match between function and biological form.

Several responses to this clash between belief systems and evolutionary biology are therefore possible. The first is angry rejection of evolutionary biology despite the extraordinary evidence that objectively overrides such an attitude. The second is to seek a compromise between two apparently very different perspectives, most often by suggesting that a deity created the natural laws through which evolution acts, or by suggesting that religion and belief in the supernatural on one hand, and science and its demonstration of evolutionary biology on the other, are different domains that do not have the capacity to inform each other. These are both positions that distinguished evolutionary and molecular scientists such as Francis Collins (one of the founders of the human genome project) and Stephen Jay Gould (the influential evolutionary biologist and science writer) have taken. The third position is to consider that supernatural belief and religion themselves are the consequences or side effects of the evolution of human consciousness and social complexity, and thus have no fundamental validity as explanations of human origins. This view has been a major plank in the rise of rationalism as a philosophical approach. It is not necessary for an understanding and application of evolutionary biology to take a personal position regarding these competing world views, except for rejecting the first approach which denies anything but a purely deistic control of all components of a species' design and creation: this attitude would deny the importance of science to medicine.

The broad philosophical implications of his discoveries were apparent to Darwin himself, and indeed inspired him to delay publishing his findings for several decades. He had been brought up in the tradition of natural theology, which viewed species as being designed by a deity to match the niches in which they lived. Although initially enamoured of this idea, it did not survive his experiences as a field researcher on the 5-year around-the-globe voyage of HMS *Beagle*. The concept that species are not immutable had been proposed before Darwin, and indeed his grandfather Erasmus Darwin had himself postulated such an idea. What Darwin and Wallace provided was a mechanistic explanation which provided for both species transmutation and for the emergence of apparent adaptive 'design' that required no external hand or designer. The subsequent development of evolutionary biology has built on these concepts, provided the detail, added molecular explanations and uncovered an extraordinary amount of empirical evidence. But as in any area of biology, there will always of course be some debate over detail and the relative importance of particular processes.

Evolutionary biology is a particularly difficult area of academic research, in no small part because of the range of disciplines it must embrace, from the most molecular to the mathematical, and it has a broad dependence on comparative approaches. The dimension of time creates particular difficulties, given that evolution is primarily dealing with change over long periods which cannot be directly observed. Particularly with respect to evolution in organisms more complex than bacteria, empirical data are difficult to obtain because of the generation times required. In the case of human evolution, research approaches are largely restricted to the interpretation of retrospective analyses. By the very nature of this approach there are often limited data sets and the interpretation may have a speculative element. A potential danger is to consider only an adaptive explanation for a trait when other possibilities also exist and need to be considered. This matter is considered further in section 2.4.4. However, despite these difficulties, the body of empirical observation from diverse species gives a very solid basis for understanding evolutionary medicine. Further, progress in molecular evolution, whereby interpretation of genomic structure can be used to rebuild lineages, has greatly overcome these practical difficulties.

Box 2.1   The origins of evolutionary thought

The beginnings of modern evolutionary thought, that species might not be fixed, appeared at the end of the eighteenth century. These concepts did not emerge in isolation but were inherently linked to the new wave of philosophical ideas and of natural science that appeared in seventeenth and eighteenth century Europe. The biologists of the eighteenth century started to see order in nature, particularly with the development of classification systems such as those of Carl Linnaeus (1707–1778), who wanted to define the divinely inspired and directed natural world with each species the subject of a separate design and creation, but later was to suggest that many species had arisen following the creation though hybridization from primal

species. The other great classifier, Georges-Louis Leclerc, Comte de Buffon (1707–1788), was far more controversial in that he was among the first to suggest that humans had emerged from a former more primitive state. Buffon also suggested some vague notion of organic evolution, alluding to the possible common ancestry of humans and the apes.

The first recognized transmutationists were Erasmus Darwin (1731–1802) and Jean-Baptiste Lamarck (1744–1819). Erasmus Darwin was a doctor and Charles Darwin's grandfather. He proposed that organisms could develop towards a higher order through accumulation of experience. He viewed life as a continuous chain from the most primitive forms to humans and published these in a volume entitled *Zoonomia* in 1794. Lamarck was a professional botanist turned zoologist from minor but impoverished nobility; he managed to survive the French Revolution to achieve a professorship in the Museum of Natural History in Paris but was to end his career in an impoverished and ignominious state. Lamarck was prolific as a biological theorist but those ideas of relevance were that the most simple species emerged by spontaneous generation and new species then emerged by progress up a ladder of development. He proposed two laws. The first was that use enhances and disuse atrophies an organ. The second law was that the effects of use or disuse were passed by reproduction to the next generation, a concept frequently referred to by a slogan, the 'inheritance of acquired characteristics'. His ideas are found in *Philosophie Zoologique* (1809), which was not well received, particularly by his influential Parisian rival Georges Cuvier (1769–1832) who was a great comparative anatomist. Both were professors of Natural History in Paris. Cuvier made major contributions to early palaeontology, being the first to unequivocally show that species became extinct: up to that time it was generally believed that species did not go extinct and that the large fossil bones found in Europe belonged to species still extant in Africa. Cuvier showed unequivocally that this was not the case and argued that most species that had ever lived were now extinct, destroyed in various catastrophic events: this was the school of 'catastrophism'. He was highly sceptical that species could change – rather, they went extinct – and his ideas were highly influential in the opposition to evolutionary concepts even after his death. The third key member of the Paris natural history professorship was Étienne Geoffroy Saint-Hilaire (1771–1844), who had developed a concept of a species transmutability somewhat similar to that of Lamarck. His lasting contribution was to demonstrate homologies between organs such as fins and limbs across phyla. He recognized the homology between the middle ear bones of mammals and the jaw bones of fishes. Some of Lamarck's ideas persisted in various ways and Darwin accepted that

inheritance of acquired characteristics may play some role in evolutionary processes. Superficially, some have suggested that modern developmental concepts contain echoes of Lamarck. This is a gross misunderstanding: Lamarck was focused on the inheritance of acquired characteristics, whereas modern epigenetic inheritance focuses on how environmental effects in one generation can affect the offspring through changes in maternal physiology and through secondary changes in gene expression in the next.

Other ideas of transmutation emerged but no credible mechanism to explain how a species might transform was presented until the work of Darwin and Wallace. By the time Darwin's book appeared the public were ready, in that an earlier popular book, *Vestiges of the Natural History of Creation*, published anonymously in 1844 but written by the Scottish journalist Robert Chambers, argued for evolution towards humanity under a divine guidance. It was highly controversial and had had great impact in that it suggested that there had been no special creation of humans, rather they were part of some continuity with lower animals.

This gradually emergent new view of biology could not be isolated from changed understandings about other aspects of the natural world. It was a changed understanding of geology that was to be so influential. A new world view, namely that the world was old and had been moulded by the gradual actions of forces such as water and ice, emerged to replace catastrophic theories, particularly that of a biblical flood. The most influential of the geologists was to be Charles Lyell, whose three volumes of *Principles of Geology* (1830–1833) and friendship heavily influenced Darwin. Indeed, Darwin's first significant scientific writings were on the emergence of coral reefs and atolls where he developed concepts which are largely valid today. Lyell, while a deist, more than any other was responsible for the new world view that the natural world was old and that change occurred slowly. He argued that the study of processes still observable was key to understanding the past and thus geological change was slow: this uniformitarian approach was in marked distinction to the catastrophic school. He was a close friend and strong supporter of Darwin, but had trouble reconciling his own religious beliefs with Darwin's concepts.

Charles Darwin was born in 1808 and came from a wealthy country background. Like his father and grandfather he was intended to be a doctor, but in Edinburgh found medicine to his dislike and biology to be his passion. One of Charles Darwin's early teachers at University in Edinburgh was Robert Grant (1793–1874), who was a committed Lamarckian and a close friend of Geoffroy Saint-Hilaire. Darwin became an enthusiastic biologist under the mentorship of Grant, studying sponges and other marine organisms and these were the subjects of Darwin's first scientific presentations. Later, Darwin was to earn, in his own mind, the credibility of being a true biologist by undertaking a decade-long study of the classification of barnacles. Not wanting to progress in medicine he moved to Cambridge, where he intended to prepare for the Church but instead became immersed in the excitement of the emerging natural sciences of geology, botany and zoology. Famously he was asked to be companion to Fitzroy on the voyage of HMS *Beagle*. He started out on that voyage in 1831 as a firm believer in natural theology as exemplified in William Paley's writings, but was to return 5 years later with his ideas of speciation and evolution starting to consolidate. There has been much written on how his ideas formed during this voyage: he recognized the relationship between fossil species in one geographical area and extant species, eventually rationalizing that they must be related over time. He recognized the power of Lyell's uniformitarian approach. Concepts of adaptive radiation were to emerge, at least in retrospect, from the specimens he had collected in his brief visit to the Galápagos Islands. His observations of the three Tierra Del Fuegians that Fitzroy was returning to Tierra Del Fuego influenced his thinking about the origins of humans and humanity. Supported by family wealth, he married his cousin

Emma and retreated to Down House in Kent to become a gentleman naturalist and biological theorist. He had already started working with breeders of pigeons and domestic animals to understand what he was to term 'artificial selection' when his reading in 1838 of Thomas Malthus's *An Essay on the Principle of Population* (the sixth edition was published in 1826) gave him the basis for insights into natural selection. Many years passed between his first consolidated notes on what we now term evolution and natural selection, which he first wrote up in an unpublished essay in 1842. Nervous of their reception, he did not present his ideas publicly until 1858 when it was read in conjunction with Alfred Wallace's paper to the Linnaean Society. A year later he was to publish the first of six editions of *The Origin of Species*. There was wide public interest in Charles Darwin's writings; his early travelogue about his travels on the Beagle had already been highly popular.

The publication of *The Origin* led to satire, parody and debate, both scientific and popular, but the issues were much deeper. The challenge of evolutionary thought was that it replaced concepts of divine order with a focus on biological materialism and determinism. Did it devalue culture? While in the early years after Darwin's work was published the debate focused largely on the issues of the role of the divine, others such as the social philosopher Herbert Spencer hijacked the Darwinian paradigm to advance issues of politics and social change. We see that these issues remain in how evolutionary sciences are understood and perceived today, particularly in North America.

The most well-known confrontation was at the British Association for the Advancement of Science meeting in Oxford in 1860 where Samuel Wilberforce, Bishop of Oxford, and Thomas Henry Huxley, Darwin's most strident supporter, had an interchange. While accounts of the meeting differ, the most widely told anecdote is that Wilberforce asked Huxley whether he was descended from monkeys on his grandfather's side or his grandmother's side, Huxley muttered: 'The Lord has delivered him into my hands' and replied that he 'would rather be descended from an ape than from a cultivated man who used his gifts of culture and eloquence in the service of prejudice and falsehood'.

The Origin was meant as an abstract of a much longer and never-completed book. Darwin's major contributions are described throughout this book and include those of natural and sexual selection; the importance of variation and heritability; and the importance of cumulative small change in the transmutation of species. These were remarkable ideas in a time when no mechanism for inheritance existed, and Darwin himself had to generate a – somewhat strange – model to explain inheritance. Darwin was much aware of the controversy his work had created. But when he died in 1882 he was buried in Westminster Abbey.

Alfred Wallace had a very different background, coming from an impoverished family, self-taught through the London Mechanics Institute, and working for many years as a commercial collector in the Amazon and South-east Asia, seeking specimens for wealthy private collectors. His recognition of the Wallace line that indicates the geographical separation between Asian and Australian fauna was the founding point for the science of biogeography. He corresponded with Darwin on issues of speciation in the 1850s. Famously, he had a very similar idea to that of natural selection, also influenced by reading Lyell and Malthus, while on the island of Ternate in the Malay Archipelago in 1858. He wrote his ideas in a letter to Darwin and Darwin was shocked to find that his unpublished idea of selection had been discovered independently. Hooker and Lyell arranged for a joint paper, entitled *On the Tendency of Species to Form Varieties; and on the Perpetuation of Varieties and Species by Natural Means of Selection* to be read to a meeting of the Linnean Society on 1 July 1858. Wallace's and Darwin's ideas were not identical in some aspects: Wallace focused on environmental change whereas Darwin understood the importance of individual variation; Wallace saw competition as being between species, Darwin between individuals. As well as becoming a social activist, Wallace became a spiritualist and developed a teleological view that the universe existed to support the evolution of the human spirit. The latter was a distinct creation from that of consciousness and that of organic matter, each of which had required some unseen supernatural spirit. Notwithstanding these ideas, which damaged Wallace's reputation and disappointed Darwin, he received many honours from the scientific community.

After this initial wave of conceptual breakthroughs, Darwinian concepts became progressively marginalized in the late nineteenth and early twentieth centuries. This eclipse of Darwinism arose from many sources. Evolution itself, that is the mutability of species, was no longer questioned except from religious quarters; the issue was the mechanism. Selection was not seen to be adequate to explain the natural world. Lamarckian arguments came back into vogue (neo-Lamarckism) both from a philosophical and scientific perspective and were to persist in the work of Lysenko (see Chapter 4 in this volume) well into the twentieth century. Other arguments were highly teleological, such as the school of orthogenesis, whose proponents wished to see a direction to evolution and play down adaptive processes.

The initial discoveries of mutations following the rediscovery of genetics led to an intense argument as to whether mutation or selection was the source of new features and new species. William Bateson, one of the earliest and most influential geneticists, was firmly of the view that saltations (that is, undirected mutations) were the real cause of evolution and that selection played no role. Thomas Morgan, the greatest of the early *Drosophila* geneticists, was also a firm saltationist but later he was to accept that external factors might influence the reproductive success of an organism carrying a mutated gene. There was a parallel set of arguments between the school of biometricians, the most prominent of whom was Darwin's cousin Francis Galton. There was a deep clash between them and the geneticists at many levels. The issue was, could the new Mendelian science, biometry and concepts of selection be reconciled? Was evolution about saltatory leaps or gradualism, and did adaptation and selection play a role?

There was great debate, eventually settled by biometricians, particularly Ronald Fisher in Cambridge. The work of Fisher, JBS Haldane and Sewall Wright all focused on population genetics and provided the mathematical and theoretical basis for the growing recognition of the compatibility of modern genetics and evolutionary thought. Because of their influence evolutionary biology was and is still heavily dominated by quantitative population genetics, a topic largely omitted from this book. By the mid-twentieth century, an influx of biologists from Russia and Europe, led by Thomas Dobzhansky and Ernst Mayr, brought a naturalist's perspective. Palaeontologists such as George Gaylord Simpson documented macroevolution and showed how it was compatible with shorter-term microevolutionary processes. By 1953, when DNA's structure was revealed, there was no gap between the ideas of genetics and the ideas of evolutionary biology. This process of integration was termed the Modern Synthesis, or neo-Darwinism.

Evolutionary biology continued to evolve and still does. The important contributions from subsequent thought leaders such as William Hamilton, Robert Trivers, EO Wilson, John Maynard Smith, Stephen Jay Gould, Richard Lewontin, and Richard Dawkins are referred to elsewhere in this book. But the issues that first provoked unease remain; here is a science that directly affects our views on human nature and behaviour and our relationships to each other and the natural world (see Chapter 12). Inevitably such a science will challenge belief systems and ideologies. But perhaps most uncomfortable of all, the idea that there is a continuum between animal social behaviours and human concepts of morality has been the biggest barrier for some.

The argument, common among creationists, that much is uncertain in evolutionary biology reflects a misunderstanding of how science works. Evolutionary science is no different than any other mainstream field of biology or medical research: the core elements are well established, while debates and competing viewpoints drive the field to address new hypotheses with new research methods. As any science progresses, there are still frontiers where more research is needed and where the relative merits of one view versus another remain to be resolved. An analogy would be a disease such as type 2 diabetes mellitus. No one would debate the role of insulin resistance in its aetiology, but there remains considerable uncertainty as to the ultimate underlying pathogenic mechanisms. For example, what are the relative roles of genetic and/or epigenetic factors and of lifestyle? Is the primary defect in the pathway of insulin's action or in pancreatic β cell function, and what is the role of vascular endothelial dysfunction or inflammatory cytokines? Similarly, there will be different views among health professionals about the optimal treatment approaches for certain individuals. But all this intense debate does not prevent a consensus about the basic pathophysiology. In this sense, then, uncertainty and debate are features of all healthy sciences, and evolutionary biology and medicine are no exception. In the case of evolutionary biology, the scientific debates are complicated by the fact that they not only have intellectual implications but also societal and religious consequences. Again, an analogy might be between orthodox views of the role of insulin and dietary control in diabetes therapy compared with the views of those who reject orthodox medical approaches in favour of faith healing.

2.2 What does evolutionary theory explain?

Everyone is familiar with the wide variety of life forms on our planet – microbial, plant and animal – which we call the biosphere. Nearly 2 million living species have been named so far, and it is estimated that there are perhaps

10–50 million extant species. These numbers are dwarfed by estimates of the number of species that have become extinct: probably only one in 1000 of species that have ever lived are still alive. Of these, a scant 250 000 or so have been preserved as fossils.

The diversity between species can appear great – compare a whale and a beetle – or small – compare two species of bacteria. Evolutionary theory provides an explanation for how this huge diversity of present and past life forms arose from ancestral species. Evolutionary theory is concerned with the diversification of life on Earth, but does not attempt to provide an explanation for *how* life originally arose, which remains an important but separate question.

Box 2.2 The origins of life

The origins of life have been the subject of much cosmological, biological and philosophical speculation, and nothing can be definitive. It has been suggested that the first replicators must have been inorganic crystals, a role later taken over by the nucleic acids. The source of energy driving replication may have been the sun but it may also have been the heat from the Earth's core: the latter is of increasing potential validity given the increasing knowledge of thermophile bacteria which live in extreme heat and make use of hydrogen sulphide. The sources of the DNA, RNA and high-energy phosphate bonds and amino acids are even more speculative. The famous experiments of Urey and Miller trying to replicate the primeval environment resulted in the formation of several amino acids from a primitive carboniferous atmosphere containing methane and ammonia. Others have suggested that carbonaceous meteorites were the source of the earliest organic molecules, including amino acids, but that just shifts the cosmic location of some initial synthesis.

A generally held hypothesis is that RNA replication evolved before DNA replication, and that RNA replication may have been autocatalytic. Indeed, it has been reported that under the right circumstances RNA can be formed from precursor molecules *in vitro* provided a catalytic enzyme is present, but then the question becomes what is the source of the initial catalyst. This RNA world is highly speculative. The lack of a double-helix capacity in contrast to DNA means its replication is much more error-prone and mutation rates are much higher. Thus, only simple viruses with small genomes are able to use RNA as their replicator. But RNA can take on tertiary structures that may allow it to be catalytic before that role was adopted by proteinaceous enzymes. From this RNA world, possessing autocatalysis and replication plus the coding of primitive proteins, may have evolved the capacity to synthesize DNA.

DNA sequence data has allowed estimation of the points of divergence between the lineages of the organisms, including plants, fungi, animals and prokaryotes, extant today. The common precursor to all forms of life lived about 3 billion years ago, and the earliest fossil evidence of bacteria is dated to about 3.5 billion years ago, the age of the earliest stromatolites, which are still formed by some cyanobacteria. The organization of the prokaryotic kingdoms is complex and uncertain, probably reflecting horizontal transfer of genes between emergent species. Two major groupings are recognized: the Archaea, which includes many anaerobic organisms living in extreme environments, and the Bacteria, which includes the bacteria with which we are traditionally familiar. The major classes of bacteria diverged perhaps 3.6 billion years ago. The origin of the Earth itself dates to about 4.5 billion years.

The first eukaryote evolved between 2.7 and 1.5 billion years ago. The origin of the nucleus in a eukaryotic cell (a cell with a nucleus) is uncertain, but sequence data suggest that it is most likely to have resulted from the engulfing of an archaeal micro-organism, which ultimately formed the nucleus, by a bacterium. Hence the human genome is more closely related to the Archaea than to the Bacteria.

Mitochondria evolved following the engulfment of another form of bacterium, probably related to the rickettsia, a process known as endosymbiosis. Chloroplasts in plant cells also arose by endosymbiosis of a cyanobacterium.

The first vertebrates evolved some 525 million years ago, whereas it was only about 640 million years ago that the first multicellular organisms appeared. Dinosaurs (and their descendants, birds)

along with other classes of reptile diverged from the lineage which was to lead to mammals some 350 million years ago and the large dinosaurs emerged between 250 and 300 million years ago. Some 70–80 million years ago all species of extant primate shared a common ancestor and placental mammals including marsupials shared a common ancestor as recently as about 110 million years ago, whereas monotremes shared a common ancestor with birds and reptiles some 300 million years ago. Figure 2.1 illustrates these evolutionary relationships.

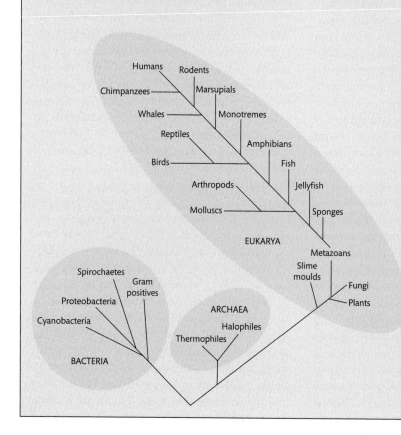

Figure 2.1 The tree of life: evolutionary relationships in the biosphere.

Evolutionary theory makes much use of the concept of adaptations, meaning features that make an organism better able to survive and reproduce and its offspring survive to reproduce in the environment in which it lives.

Such adaptations may sometimes give the impression that an organism has been 'designed' for its environment. Yet as we will see below, evolutionary theory is able to explain adaptation to an environment by invoking a rather simple process of natural selection – differential survival and subsequent reproduction – acting on genetic variation within a breeding population.

How can we tell that an organism is well adapted to its environment; that is, better able to survive and reproduce? What could be the measure of such ability? The measure used by evolutionary biologists is **fitness**, the potential for an individual (strictly, its genotype, although of course it is the phenotype which is mating) to survive and reproduce: a function of its **reproductive success** or the number of reproducing offspring it produces. If a particular genotype in a population increases in frequency in the next generation relative to the average frequency of all genotypes in that population then that genotype has greater fitness. For example, if under a particular set of selective conditions an individual (for simplicity we will use an example of an asexually reproducing organism) produces three viable offspring whereas all other individuals in the population produce only two viable offspring, then the **relative fitness** of that individual is 1.5 and the proportion of that genotype in the population will increase by 50% in the next generation. It is important to remember that fitness is measured in a particular environment, and a genotype with greater fitness in one environment may be inferior to another genotype when placed in a different environment.

We have considered the simple example of the **direct fitness** of an individual organism that reproduces by asexual reproduction. Of course, for sexual reproduction the fitness of each parent must be considered: this brings into play considerations of mating success and sexual selection, and these will be considered in more detail below. Beyond the direct fitness of individual parents, we must remember that an individual shares components of their genotype with their close relatives, and any action by an individual which improves the reproductive success (i.e. direct fitness) of a close relative will consequently improve the **indirect fitness** of that individual by ensuring that at least some of those shared **alleles** (one of the different forms of a gene that can occur at a specific locus on a chromosome) will be transmitted to the next generation. The sum of direct and indirect fitness is called **inclusive fitness**, and we will consider the social and behavioural aspects of optimizing inclusive fitness below and in Chapter 10.

2.3 How does evolution work?

Charles Darwin described evolution as 'descent with modification'. Here, descent refers to the common ancestry of all species, and modification refers to the various changes that occurred in the descendants of these ancestors as they adapted to new and changing environments. In more modern terminology, we now accept the insights of Darwin and Wallace that evolution occurs because of the following mechanisms and processes (Figure 2.2).

- Species tend to produce more offspring than the resources available can support.
- Individual members of a species vary in ways that affect their ability to compete for resources (**variation**).
- Some subset of this variation is heritable (**inheritance**).
- Differential survival and reproduction among these variant forms leads to over-representation of successful forms in the next generation (**selection**).
- Selection over generations leads to change in the composition of the population (**evolution**).

It is important to understand that evolution operates on populations of organisms over generations. Individual organisms do not evolve during their lifetime: they may be able to change some aspects of their **phenotype** in response to the environment (a process known as **plasticity** which is discussed in Chapter 4) but those changes are not heritable and are not passed on to their offspring (there may be some exceptions to this rule for epigenetic changes in developmental plasticity; see Chapter 4). Although natural selection operates at the individual level through favouring particular characteristics (**traits**) in the phenotype which contribute to improved survival or reproductive success, for a population to evolve those phenotypic traits must be associated with heritable factors in the genotype to ensure that the selected trait is passed on to the next generation. In other words, selection must result in changes in allele frequencies in the gene(s) that determine those traits.

In the following sections we look at the processes of variation, selection, and inheritance in more detail.

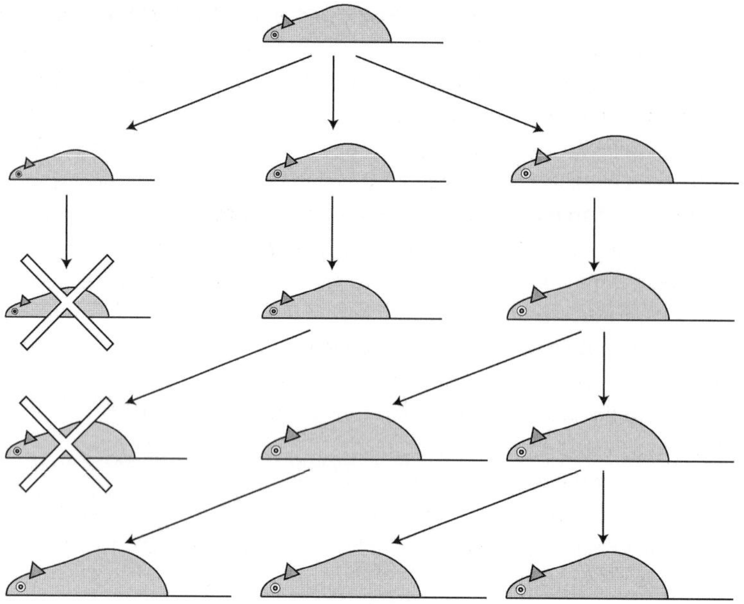

Figure 2.2 Evolution operates through processes of variation followed by selection causing differential survival or reproductive ability.

2.3.1 Variation

Before Darwin, biologists were enthusiastic classifiers; indeed, Darwin himself spent many years classifying barnacles. The system of classification invented by Carl Linnaeus in the eighteenth century relied on shared physical characteristics to place organisms into orders, families, genera and species, with a nominated specimen (the type specimen) considered as the standard for identification of other members of the species. The focus was therefore on establishing *similarities* between individuals of a species. But the work of Darwin emphasized the importance of *variation* among individuals of that species as the raw material for selective mortality and reproductive success, allowing populations gradually to change their numbers of different variants over time. If there is no variation between individuals in a population there are no discriminatory traits for selection to act on and, therefore, no capacity for evolution to take place. We can easily appreciate how widely organisms from the same species can vary: humans, who along with the domestic dog represent one of the more variable of mammalian species, vary markedly both in physical appearance – height, build, skin, hair, and eye colour – and in less obvious characteristics such as blood group, tissue type, lactase expression, and disease susceptibility. There is no physical type specimen for *H. sapiens* and recent genomic data has underlined that there is no type specimen for the human genome either. Examination of other species by morphological and molecular methods also reveals wide variation among individuals.

What is the source of this variation among individuals in a population? The principal sources of heritable (genetic) variation – genetic novelty – are **mutation** and (in sexually reproducing organisms) **recombination**. Additionally, as we discuss in more detail in Chapter 4, environmental factors during the development of an individual can modify the phenotype by the process called **developmental** (or **phenotypic**) **plasticity**; the ability of developmental processes to generate phenotypic novelty for selection to act on has become an important topic in evolutionary developmental biology in recent years.

2.3.1.1 Mutation

A mutation is a change in the base pairs in the DNA sequence, and therefore by definition it is heritable as long as it occurs in the **germ line**. So a somatic mutation which occurred in a population of dividing cells in the body, for example in the intestinal mucosa, might have a dramatic effect on those cells (it could produce a tumour) but clearly cannot be passed to the next generation. Here we are concerned only with *heritable* changes. The scale of such possible changes ranges from a single base substitution, giving rise to a **single nucleotide polymorphism** or SNP, through duplication of blocks of tens to thousands of base pairs (a process resulting in so-called **variable numbers of tandem repeats** or VNTRs), to deletion, duplication, or inversion of whole genes or gene-sized blocks of non-coding DNA. Larger changes compatible with life, such as duplication or deletion of whole chromosomes (**aneuploidy**), are not infrequent but cannot be passed on to the next generation. The molecular basis of mutation is discussed in Chapter 3.

Because a new mutation typically affects only one copy of DNA, individuals carrying a new mutation, or their offspring, will be **heterozygous** for that mutation. The consequences of the mutation will depend on a number of factors, such as whether it occurs in a coding or non-coding region of the genome and whether its phenotypic effect – if it has one, for as explained in Chapter 3 many mutations are phenotypically silent – is **dominant** or **recessive**. The existence of silent and recessive mutations suggests that hidden variation is common in the genome; indeed, most single-base substitutions are thought to be selectively neutral or only mildly deleterious and do not significantly affect the fitness of the carrier. This of course also means that they will be passed on to the next generation.

Mutations arise either from physical damage to DNA by factors such as chemical mutagens or ionizing radiation, or from errors in the DNA replication (copying) process during mitosis or meiosis. The rate of mutation can be estimated from laboratory experiments with simple organisms, or for more complex organisms by comparing the DNA sequences of related species for which there is phylogenetic evidence about the time of divergence. Rates of single-base substitution are low, of the order of $(1-2) \times 10^{-8}$ per base pair per generation for eukaryotes.

Yet, because of the size of the genome (about 6.5×10^9 base pairs for humans, of which 2.5% is expected to be 'functional'), one or two new base substitutions are estimated to occur in each functional human diploid genome per generation. Rates of formation of VNTRs are more difficult to measure but appear to be higher than for single-base substitutions.

Studies of human genetic disease (see Chapter 3) suggest that rates of mutation vary according to parental age and sex, with an approximately 10-fold excess of new disease-associated mutations being of paternal origin. During oogenesis, all of the 23 cell divisions necessary to produce a woman's lifelong complement of oocytes occur before she is born. In males, who produce sperm throughout life after puberty, 36 germ-line cell divisions occur before puberty and approximately 23 every year thereafter, so that a sperm from a 35-year-old man is the product of about 500 cell divisions. The greater number of cell divisions over a longer time span provides greater mutational opportunity.

The British biologist JBS Haldane was the first to estimate mutation rates in humans from a study in 1935 of the prevalence of the blood-clotting defect haemophilia (an X-linked recessive disorder, therefore occurring in all male carriers) in British men. Since at that time haemophilia almost completely prevented fertility in affected men, Haldane reasoned that under conditions of unchanging prevalence most new cases must arise by mutation, and the mutation rate for that gene on the X chromosome per generation would be approximately one-third of the prevalence rate (since females have two X chromosomes and males have one). Haldane's estimate of 2×10^{-5} mutations per allele per generation proved to be remarkably accurate, fitting well with the estimate quoted above of $(1-2) \times 10^{-8}$ mutations per base pair per generation (since an average protein-coding gene will consist of about 1000 base pairs).

2.3.1.2 Recombination

Sexually reproducing organisms inherit their parents' genes, not their genotypes (or their phenotypes). This is because of the genetic variation introduced by two processes during sexual reproduction: first, meiosis during gametogenesis involves recombination, exchange of genetic material between pairs of homologous chromosomes, and secondly the fusion of the two gametes, each with a parental haploid genome.

The process of recombination can generate high levels of variation in offspring because it generates new combinations of alleles on a chromosome. This is particularly likely to have an effect on the phenotype if the genes affected have additive or subtractive effects on some trait. For example, consider four genes all determining a trait such as susceptibility to a particular disease, with alleles A, B, C, and D each independently increasing susceptibility by the same amount and alleles a, b, c, and d independently decreasing susceptibility by that amount. The parental genotypes might be AbCd and aBcD, each with moderate susceptibility, but recombination during gametogenesis might produce gametes with genotypes ABCD and abcd, with the potential to confer high and low disease susceptibility, respectively, on offspring receiving those genotypes (see Chapter 3).

2.3.1.3 Constraints on variation

Constraints on variation may explain why organisms often show examples of poor 'design'. They appear not to be as ideally suited to their environment as they could be.

Why should variation be constrained? There are a number of reasons, which as we will see in later chapters may explain some aspects of human disease. First, at least in multicellular organisms, accumulation of genetic variation and its testing by selection are slow processes, so that response to a new selective pressure such as environmental change will also be slow. As we will discuss in later chapters, this lag time may lead to a mismatch between an organism and its environment if environmental change is faster than evolutionary processes, set by the naturally occurring rate of generation of new variants. A second constraint occurs because evolution by variation and selection demands continuous 'improvement' and does not permit partial dismantling of an existing variant of modest fitness (with the effect of reducing fitness in intermediate generations) in order to construct a better solution (Figure 2.3). An example of this effect is the human eye. The eye has an adequate, but flawed design, which routes nerves and blood vessels over the top of the retinal photoreceptors (Figure 2.4), but it is improbable that it could evolve towards the octopus eye (where the retina faces the 'right' way) without passing through a non-functional and non-adaptive form.

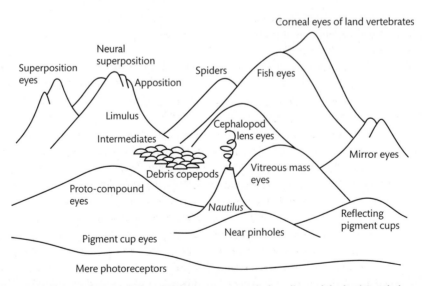

Figure 2.3 An adaptive landscape of eye evolution. Height represents optical quality and the horizontal plane represents evolutionary distance. An eye can evolve 'uphill', as its fitness increases continuously, but cannot evolve from one peak to another as to do so would require traversing a valley of lower fitness (from Dawkins, R. (1996) *Climbing Mount Improbable.* Norton, New York; figure originally drawn by Professor Michael Land, University of Sussex).

our genes and thus are also capable of passing these on to their descendants; our cousins share a quarter of our genes, and so forth. Thus we can improve our fitness, since it is defined by the successful passage of our genes to subsequent reproducing generations, by encouraging our close relatives to reproduce. Inclusive fitness is the term used to describe this concept; that is, the impact of a given allele on both the carrier's own fitness and that of neighbours or relatives carrying the same allele. The assumption is then that individuals act not only to maximize their individual fitness but their inclusive fitness: within families this is the process of kin selection. As JBS Haldane put it, 'I would be prepared to lay down my life for two brothers or eight cousins!'

Kin selection can explain the evolution of altruism because it develops in social animals such as insects in which there is a high degree of relatedness between the individuals. The haplodiploid nature of bee genetics, whereby females are diploid and males are haploid, means that female workers share up to three-quarters of their genes with the queen's other female offspring, more than the 50% they could share with their own offspring were they able to mate. This could explain why it is in their evolutionary interest to forego reproducing themselves but to support the survival of the queen's offspring. Similarly in humans or in other mammals living in small groups, siblings have a high genetic relatedness with each other's offspring, and an individual's genes can be transmitted to future generations not only by promoting the reproductive fitness of his or her own offspring but also by promoting the fitness of their nieces and nephews. We shall leave to Chapter 7 considering the additive (and complicating) role of uncertain paternity in primate social structures.

However, the evolution of altruism does not necessarily require a group-selective explanation: reciprocal cooperation may lead to behaviour which can be interpreted as altruism. There is advantage in cooperating in situations where A is more likely to help B if B had helped A in the past. As there may be situations where help is essential for A to survive and reproduce, then alleles controlling cooperative behaviour will be more likely to survive and to increase in frequency. The classic example is that of the vampire bat, where a bat will provide blood to a hungry yet unrelated bat in the same colony. Even so, vampire bats are sensitive to which animals have and have

not shared meals in the past, weeding out any would-be cheaters. This is not group selection but selection for a form of delayed self-interest that benefits an individual's fitness, since the cost to a bat of sharing food is offset by its expectation that it will benefit from reciprocal behaviour in the future. There is an extensive literature in game theory to identify how competition and poor cooperation can be dealt with through the evolution of policing, reciprocation and punishment, leading to evolutionarily stable strategies, and this will be discussed in Chapter 10 with respect to its implications for understanding human behaviour.

2.3.2.5 Genes as units of selection

Implicit in the discussion above is the notion that selection *acts on* the phenotype and eventually *benefits* the organism's lineage by matching its phenotype to the environment. For instance, in a species subject to the pressure of predation, selection might result in adaptation at the level of the individual, such as a change in muscle biochemistry allowing faster escape, or perhaps at the level of the group, such as a change in behaviour whereby some individuals reduce their apparent individual fitness by acting as sentinels to warn the group of the presence of a predator.

A different perspective was provided by Richard Dawkins with his important concept of the **selfish gene**. While not denying that selection acts on the phenotype, Dawkins argued that the ultimate beneficiary of adaptation is the gene itself, in that genes are the agents which over the long term survive, or fail to survive, because of the benefits they confer, or the limitations they impose, on the phenotypes that they generate. In this view, genes are considered as the permanent 'replicators' and phenotypes as the temporary, generation-based 'vehicles', formed by coalitions of genes, that they inhabit. Even the genotype can be considered as temporary, as in sexually reproducing species it is destroyed in each generation by meiosis and recombination. The selfish-gene metaphor therefore characterizes an adaptation as something which increases the ability of a gene to promote its own survival without necessarily promoting the survival of the organism, group or even species. Most commonly, of course, the interests of a gene and its 'vehicle' (the organism) do coincide, but they may not. An example was mentioned above, where an individual organism reduces its own fitness – limits its foraging time and increases its preda-tion risk – by acting as a sentinel. This apparently unself-ish behaviour can be explained from the selfish gene's viewpoint by considering a closely related group who share many alleles. By protecting other group members from predation, the sentinel is helping to ensure survival of its genes – even though they happen to be residing in other members of the group. As recognized by William Hamilton (see above, and discussion of Hamilton's rule in Chapter 7), the degree of relatedness should deter-mine the extent of such altruistic effort. Hamilton further suggested that alleles that were somehow able to 'signal' their presence in an individual would be at an advantage in triggering altruistic behaviour toward that individual from other individuals carrying the same allele.

More extreme examples of genes acting 'selfishly' can be found in the various phenomena collectively known as **intragenomic conflict**, in which genetic elements proliferate at the expense of other genes in the same genome. They may do so by ensuring that they are over-represented in the gametes, or by promiscuously copying themselves to increase their abundance in the genome. **Meiotic drive** or **segregation distortion** occurs when an allele is able to 'cheat' on the normal process of Mendelian segregation (which ensures that each of the two alleles in a diploid genome has a 50% chance of appearing in a gamete), increasing its chances of being passed on to the next generation. Segregation distortion of sex-linked genes can bias the sex ratio of the offspring. **Transposons** (see Chapter 3) are the most abundant class of selfish genetic elements that promote their own transmission by promiscuous replication.

2.3.2.6 Extended phenotype

We introduced the concept of natural selection by con-sidering a simple scenario: namely one in which an individual's fitness is solely determined by his or her phenotype. We have used phenotype as a description of the totality of an organism's behavioural and biological traits. However, the impact of the genotype can extend beyond the physical limits of the organism, and these can also have an impact on the direction and pace of evo-lution. This concept of the **extended phenotype** was a second important contribution of Richard Dawkins. The body, the phenotype, is something genes build for them-selves to make their way through the world. The extended phenotype is *everything* that the genes can influence to gain advantage. It includes the effect of social behaviour of one individual on other individuals in the population, the manipulative effects of parasites and pathogens on the behaviour or life cycle of their hosts, the creation of artefacts – spiders' webs and birds' nests – and, most spectacularly, the engineering of the environment by building structures such as termite mounds or beaver dams through niche construction. The human ability to produce material culture – from stone tools to airlin-ers – and our ability to modify our environment to suit our physiology has allowed the human species to spread across the planet. Equally, we are clearly social animals where social behaviour is both a major component of our phenotype and a major component of our select-ive environment. The ideas of extended phenotype and niche construction should not be taken to extremes: the acid test is the presence of a direct correlation between variation in the structure or behaviour and variation in the transmission of the genes responsible for that struc-ture or behaviour.

2.3.3 Inheritance

The limitation which Darwin faced in developing his ideas was that the nature of inheritance was not under-stood. Darwin himself proposed a rather bizarre model of inheritance called pangenesis, which involved accu-mulation in the gonads of so-called gemmules shed from body tissues. Nevertheless, he realized that any mechan-ism of inheritance that involved mixing or averaging of the characteristics of the parents (blending inheritance) presented a problem for his theory of descent with modification, since the advantage of any new variation would be diluted out within a few generations. It is part of the tradition of evolutionary biology that, although it was during Darwin's lifetime that Mendel made his fundamental discovery that the individual units of gen-etic information remained intact and unmixed during transmission from one generation to the next (particu-late inheritance), Mendel's findings remained unrecog-nized until the early twentieth century. They formed the basis of modern **genetics** (a term introduced by William Bateson in 1906), along with the rapid recognition of the role of the chromosome in inheritance, and in 1909 the unit of particulate inheritance was given the name gene by Wilhelm Johannsen; Johannsen also recognized that there was not a direct link between gene and trait and he coined the terms phenotype and genotype. These accumulated concepts led to the rapid application of quantitative techniques to the study of inheritance. After initial debate over whether continuous variation of a trait (as is usually observed in biology; for example, height or weight in humans) could be generated through particulate inheritance of the type described by Mendel (whose peas were dichotomously yellow or green, round or wrinkled, etc.), the matter was firmly resolved in 1918 by the great mathematical biologist Ronald Fisher, who demonstrated that Mendelian inheritance acting across *many* genes, each making a small but additive contribution to the trait, could nonetheless in combination

account for continuous variation. During this period it became clear that genetic theory and evolutionary theory were not distinct but in fact were rather tightly linked. Indeed, it was genetic biology that provided a mechanism by which the effects of selection operated. Complex models were developed and evolutionary biology became formalized in mathematical terms (which are beyond the scope of this book). Since this Modern Synthesis of evolution and genetics, a common definition of evolution is 'change in the allele frequencies within a population over time'. As we will see in Chapter 3, molecular genetic studies of allele frequencies in humans provide evidence for the selective pressures that have shaped populations in the past and continue to do so in the present.

Box 2.3   Equations of evolution

Evolutionary biology has a strong quantitative heritage. A key element in the Modern Synthesis was the contribution of biometricians showing that Mendelian genetics and natural selection were compatible concepts. Quantitative population genetics became a major component of evolutionary research. For a diploid species it is important to distinguish between the **allele frequency** (the proportion of that allele across all gene copies in the population) and the **genotype frequency** (the proportion of a population with a specific allele pair at a particular locus). It is their interdependencies and how these are defined under different conditions that is at the heart of quantitative evolutionary biology. Evolutionary change can be defined as a change in the genotype and allele frequencies from generation to generation. A change in such frequencies is taken, all else being equal, as evidence for selection. These formal models generally require a number of assumptions about the population under study which are often not met, particularly if the population is small.

The **Hardy–Weinberg equilibrium** is a simple statement of how allele frequencies in a population show stable proportionalities in a population at equilibrium (that is, not undergoing active positive or negative selection). It is based on several assumptions including that all individuals within the population can mate at random (that is there is no assortative mating or male dominance). In the simplest case of two alleles, A and a, there are three possible genotypes: AA, Aa, and aa. If the allele frequency of A is p and that of a is q, then the genotypes are distributed in each new generation as p^2, $2pq$, and q^2. Importantly, for a population in equilibrium both the genotype and allelic frequencies remain in the same ratios over successive generations. The mathematics is obviously more complex when there are multiple alleles and multiple loci involved, but the principles remain. The mathematics underlying the relationships between two loci in the Hardy–Weinberg model allow estimates of **linkage disequilibrium**; that is, the deviation of the two-locus gamete allele frequencies from the product of the respective single-locus allele frequencies and thus of measures of recombination.

It is thus possible to examine the allelic and genotype frequencies in a population of interest to see if they are compatible with the Hardy–Weinberg formula. If not then one of the assumptions has been broken: mating may not be random, the population is too small and genetic drift may be occurring, there may be migration of others into the population, or that there is a selective process conferring unequal survival/reproduction rates on some of the genotypes. This latter possibility means that if other assumptions have been dealt with, say by having a very large population to study, evidence for selection can be inferred from examining allelic and genotypic frequencies. Conversely, where the population is in equilibrium but there is a clear disadvantage to possessing the homozygous state of one allele, then it may imply that the heterozygotic state of the persisting disadvantageous allele confers a selective advantage. This is **balancing selection**: the classical example is that of heterozygous advantage in malaria resistance in carrying one allele coding for the haemoglobinopathy underlying sickle cell anaemia.

Allelic frequencies often differ between subpopulations of a species, reflecting founder effects, drift, non-random mating, or selection acting on the population. Examples of each are found within the chapters of this book. There are many mathematical techniques used in evolutionary biology to define and dissect out these different mechanisms.

The study of variation is central to evolutionary biology. It is of historical interest that **analysis of variance** techniques were first developed and used by Fisher to define and mathematically separate genetic and environmental determinants of phenotype and their interactions in artificial selection (animal breeding) experiments and to seek evidence in wild populations for natural selection. Variations may be induced by genomic, developmental (epigenetic), or environmental factors and it is clear that it is difficult if not impossible to fully separate these effects as they are highly interdependent; indeed,

much of modern evolutionary developmental biology is based on the inability to do so. However, there are obvious practical advantages in trying to understand the relative importance of these different factors in generating variation in a trait.

A key driver in early quantitative genetics was animal and plant breeding. A key question was to what extent is the variance in phenotype based on genetics. The **heritability** (generally indicated as h^2) of a trait was defined from these simple estimates of variance as the ratio of the variance due to genotype to the total phenotypic variance of the population. The most common way of estimating h^2 is to look at the regression between parental and offspring measures of the trait. If there is a high correlation it would imply a strong genetic basis for the trait and if there is no correlation then there is no genetic contribution to the variation and, from the breeder's perspective, no value in a selection programme. There are important limitations on the estimates of heritability and most of the literature assumes two sources of variation – genetic and environmental – and considers the latter largely as a noise factor. The recognition that not all that is inherited need be genetic but might be epigenetic has confounded matters and even more so has been the growing recognition of the role of developmental plasticity and the developmental environment itself (see Chapter 4). By definition h^2 is defined by examining a population in a particular context, and under different environments the observed heritability may be very different. The heritability of adult height will be very different in a population living in circumstances of food insecurity and frequent infection during childhood to those living under optimal conditions in childhood. Obviously a breeder with a plant or animal population will seek an optimal environment. Such estimates are not possible in a human. But constraints may also play a role. A plant might be selected for optimal growth and there may be a high variance in the founder population which has a high genetic components. But after generations of selection all the plants may have reached very similar heights because of some molecular level in addition to at the level of the whole organism has greatly accelerated our understanding. Equally, it is important to recognize that not every characteristic of an organism necessarily evolved for adaptive advantage. It is easy to fall into the trap of developing an adaptive argument for every characteristic: strictly, a

trait should not be termed adaptive unless it is shown to have conferred some fitness advantage. Often such proof is difficult to achieve in practical terms and assumptions must be made, but they must be made with caution. As this chapter has attempted to demonstrate, by its very nature some aspects of evolutionary theory may not be amenable to empirical enquiry. This situation is not unique – it is common to most sciences. Whereas the areas of debate are often seized upon by those whose belief systems are threatened by the science of evolution, we hope that the reader can already see that, from what we *do* know, knowledge of evolutionary principles is enormously helpful to understanding human biology in health and disease.

KEY POINTS

- Evolutionary science explains how the huge diversity of present and past life forms arose.

- Heritable variation between particular characteristics (traits) of individuals causes differential reproductive success (fitness), leading to the accumulation of beneficial variations (adaptations) in subsequent generations.

- Changes in an individual's genotype (caused by mutations or recombination) are the basis of heritable variation. For selection to act, those changes must cause differences in the phenotype.

- Selection acts on phenotypic characteristics influencing survival and reproduction (natural selection) or ability to obtain a mate (sexual selection).

- It is a fundamental principle of evolutionary medicine that selection acts to optimize reproductive success, not necessarily the health or longevity of an individual.

- Random genetic drift can influence the evolution of a species, particularly in the presence of founder effects and population bottlenecks.

- While evolution does not have a purpose or a direction there are constraints on evolutionary possibilities, including those imposed by limits on variation and by the evolutionary history of a lineage.

- Not all the characteristics of an organism need have an adaptive explanation.

- Many adaptive arguments, no matter how plausible, must remain hypothetical rather than proven. Evolutionary thinking should avoid the trap of teleology.

Further reading

Adami, C., Ofria, C. and Collier, T.C. (2000) Evolution of biological complexity. *Proceedings of the National Academy of Sciences USA* **97**, 4463–4468.

Andersson, M.B. (1994) *Sexual Selection*. Princeton University Press, Princeton, NJ.

Burt, A. and Trivers, R. (2006) *Genes in Conflict: The Biology of Selfish Genetic Elements*. Harvard University Press, Cambridge, MA.

Darwin, C.R. (1839) *The Voyage of the Beagle*. Bartelby, New York.

Darwin, C.R. (1859) *On the Origin of Species by Means of Natural Selection, or the Preservation of Favoured Races in the Struggle for Life*, 1st edn. John Murray, London.

Darwin, C.R. (1871) *The Descent of Man, and Selection in Relation to Sex*. John Murray, London.

Dawkins, R. (1976) *The Selfish Gene*. Oxford University Press, Oxford.

Dawkins, R. (1982) *The Extended Phenotype*. Oxford University Press, Oxford.

Dawkins, R. (2004) *The Ancestor's Tale A Pilgrimage To The Dawn Of Life*. Weidenfeld & Nicholson, London.

Futuyma, D.J. (2005) *Evolution*. Sinauer Associates, Sunderland, MA.

Gould, S.J. (1996) *Full House*. Harmony Books, New York.

Maynard Smith, J. and Szathmáry, E. (1995) *The Major Transitions in Evolution*. Oxford University Press, Oxford.

Odling-Smee, F.J., Laland, K.N., and Feldman, M.W. (2003) *Niche Construction: the Neglected Process in Evolution*. Princeton University Press, Princeton, NJ.

Okasha, S. (2006) *Evolution and the Levels of Selection.* Clarendon Press, Oxford.

Pigliucci, M. and Kaplan, J. (2006) *Making Sense of Evolution: the Conceptual Foundations of Evolutionary Biology.* University of Chicago Press, Chicago, IL.

Quammen, D. (2007) *The Reluctant Mr. Darwin: an Intimate Portrait of Charles Darwin and the Making of his Theory of Evolution.* WW Norton, New York.

Ruse, M. (2006) *Darwinism and Its Discontents.* Cambridge University Press, New York.

Templeton, A.R. (2006) *Population Genetics and Microevolutionary Theory.* Wiley Liss, New York.

Williams, G.C. (1996) *Adaptation and Natural Selection*, 2nd edn. Princeton University Press, Princeton, NJ.

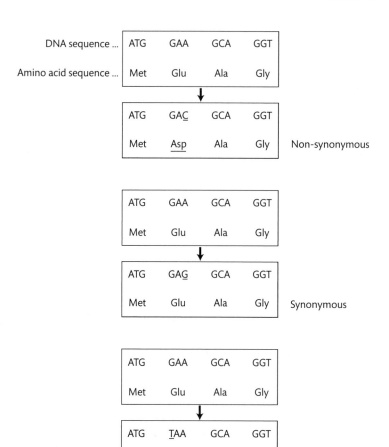

Figure 3.3 Effects of SNPs within a protein-coding region. Synonymous mutations do not change the protein sequence and are silent. Non-synonymous mutations may alter the amino acid sequence or cause premature termination of the protein sequence by insertion of a stop codon.

persistence, which is caused by one of a number of adjacent SNPs in a regulatory region some 14 000 base pairs upstream from the lactase gene itself (see Chapter 1 and Figure 3.2).

SNPs arise from two different processes: mistakes in copying the DNA sequence during replication, and chemical or physical mutagenesis caused by environmental chemicals or ionizing radiation. Although the DNA polymerase that copies DNA is extremely accurate, having an error rate of only 10^{-9} to 10^{-11} per nucleotide, each replication of the diploid genome requires copying of 6×10^9 nucleotides, suggesting that an error will occur every few replications. Similarly, although complex mechanisms have evolved to detect and repair DNA damage caused by chemical and physical mutagens, these mechanisms are also not entirely free from error.

Estimates of the effective mutation rate (the actual likelihood that a base substitution will occur at a particular site in the germ line per generation) can be made from comparison of non-functional sequences (to eliminate the effects of selection) in species whose divergence times are known. Using such an approach with human and chimpanzee sequences, a rate of base substitution of about 2×10^{-8} per site per generation was estimated. This implies that 50–100 new base substitutions (i.e. not present in the soma of either parent) will occur in the germ line per individual per generation, of which on average one or two will occur in a protein-coding region. Conversely, the low mutation rate per site and the effects of selection, drift, and past population bottlenecks together imply that any given SNP in a protein-coding region is unlikely to have arisen independently more than once during the course of human evolution (although a few examples to the contrary are known). This has two important implications for evolutionary genetic studies: first, it is reasonable to assume that if two individuals have a particular SNP, they have inherited it from a common ancestor; second, ancestral alleles, and therefore the direction of evolutionary change, can be identified from knowledge of the genome sequences of the great apes (particularly the chimpanzee, our closest living relative).

3.2.4 Indels

Indels are short insertions or deletions (most frequently one to three base pairs) within the DNA sequence. If they occur in a protein-coding region, indels are more likely to be deleterious than SNPs because they have the potential to cause insertion or deletion of one or more amino acids (if the indel is three or a multiple of three bases long) or cause frameshift mutations (if the indel is not a multiple of three bases) that may completely disrupt the production of the protein.

As with SNPs, indels are found less frequently in functional segments of the genome. Rates of mutation giving rise to indels are about 10-fold lower than those giving rise to SNPs.

The best-known example of a disease-causing indel is the three-base-pair deletion removing the phenylalanine residue at position 508 of the cystic fibrosis transmembrane conductance regulator (CFTR) protein, which is one of the mutations causing cystic fibrosis (see Box 3.3, below).

3.2.5 VNTRs

VNTRs are segments of the genome where short- to medium-length blocks of sequence are repeated in tandem arrays. The length of each repeat and the number of repeats vary widely. The length of the repeat unit of microsatellites is one to six base pairs and 10–30 repeats are typical; the repeating unit of minisatellites is up to 100 base pairs and up to 1000 repeats are possible, and satellites have repeat units of several hundred base pairs. In the longer repeats (minisatellites and satellites) the repeat units may show some variability in their sequence. VNTRs are highly variable in the number of individual repeats because they too are affected by errors during the processes of recombination and DNA replication, leading

to mutation rates (i.e. changes in the number of repeats) of up to several percentage points per generation.

Although most VNTRs are neutral, with little or no phenotypic effect, certain microsatellites are particularly dynamic and can expand rapidly in repeat number over a few generations. For example, rapid expansion of the CAG trinucleotide microsatellite within the coding region of the huntingtin gene causes Huntington's disease.

3.2.6 Transposable elements

Retrotransposons are dispersed but repetitive DNA elements that can move within the genome by a 'copy and paste' mechanism, which inserts a new copy of the element at a random site. Over 40% of the mammalian genome consists of retrotransposons, which exist at a total copy number of approximately 1.5 million, divided into classes based on size and mechanism of propagation. Many retrotransposons originated from insertion of retroviruses into the genome. Most retrotransposons are of ancient origin and have mutated to such an extent that they have lost the ability to be copied and inserted; however, several retrotransposon families are of more recent origin, some being young enough to be human-specific, and are still active in retrotransposition. Indeed, some retrotransposons have inserted into the human genome so recently that populations are polymorphic for the presence of an element at a particular chromosomal location and hence the element can be used as a genetic marker of ancestry. Individual variation in retrotransposition potential makes an important contribution to human genetic diversity.

Retrotransposons can disrupt protein-coding or regulatory regions at the site of insertion, altering gene expression and creating a disease phenotype (see Box 3.1). Retrotransposons may also have wider effects on genome structure through promoting recombination and deletion events that have evolutionary consequences. For example, a retrotransposition event caused deletion of the active-site exon of the human CMP-*N*-acetylneuraminic acid hydroxylase (CMAH) gene some 2–3 million years ago, after the divergence from our last common ancestor with chimpanzees. This causes humans to be deficient in the sialic acid *N*-glycolylneuraminic acid (Neu5Gc), which is a common constituent of cell-surface glycoproteins in other mammals, with postulated effects on pathogen resistance and brain development

The survival of this new neutral mutation will vary essentially by chance – on whether it happens to be present in a gamete that is successful in forming a member of the next generation. What happens in the next few generations depends largely on the size of the population. In a small population, random variation will cause the allele either to disappear (0% frequency in the population) or to become fixed (100% frequency in the population). Thus, small populations are more likely to be homozygous than larger populations. In a larger population, random variation is likely to maintain the allele at an intermediate frequency for a longer period, with little change in frequencies between generations, and the population will have higher levels of heterozygosity (Figure 3.6).

Population size is therefore a major predictor of the extent of genetic diversity in terms of the variation in allele frequency caused by genetic drift. But what do we mean by population size? For humans, this question is likely to elicit the answer of about 6.6 billion, the total number of humans now living. But for the purposes of estimating the extent of genetic drift, the **effective population size** is very much smaller than the actual (or census) population size. This is because simple models used to calculate drift make a number of assumptions, including no overlap between generations, constant population size over time, random mating among members of the population, and no difference in reproductive success between individuals in the population. Brief reflection shows that these assumptions are not applicable to most organisms, and especially not to humans. There is much overlap between human generations, with evolutionary consequences. The human population size has expanded at least 1000-fold within recorded history (Chapter 1). We do not mate randomly; human expansion out of Africa resulted in a number of partly isolated subpopulations within which **gene flow** was limited (at least until the establishment of modern patterns of travel and migration). The human preference for **assortative mating** (the tendency for

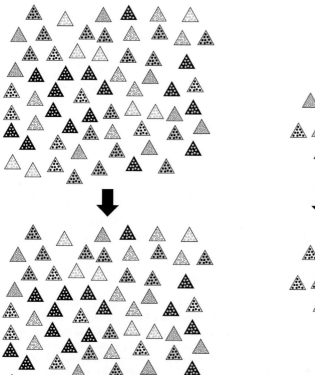

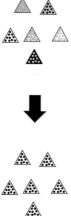

Figure 3.6 Genetic drift. In the absence of selection, allele frequencies in large populations change only slowly over generations (left). In small populations, the stochastic nature of reproductive processes means that alleles may be lost or fixed within a few generations (right).

people to choose their mates according to phenotypic similarity) further tends to reduce diversity. There is variation among individuals in reproductive success: some individuals have many children and some have few. Since that variation is unequally distributed among the sexes (being greater in men than in women; see Chapter 6), measures of drift will even vary according to whether autosomes or sex chromosomes are analysed.

The effective population size is therefore defined as the size of the idealized population (i.e. a population that conforms with the assumptions made above) that shows the same amount of genetic drift as the real-world population. Modelling shows that the factor having most influence on effective population size is often the extent of historical fluctuation in the population, with the historically smallest population sizes having the largest effect. There have been many estimates of the total effective population size of humans, using various genetic markers, and the results are always in the thousands rather than the billions, showing that the present extent of human diversity reflects expansion from a small population in the past. Note that although the discussion above uses the total human population as an example, these arguments can be applied to any identifiable subpopulation. Indeed, comparisons of the diversity (effective population size) of worldwide subpopulations can provide valuable evidence about the history and origin of different human groups.

Because of these considerations, the effective population size is not equivalent to the actual number of individuals in a population. For example, estimates of the effective population size involved in peopling the Americas are in the range of 100–200, but this does not mean that only that number of individuals were actually involved in migration across Beringia some 10 000 to 15 000 years ago (see Chapter 6).

Two important reasons for reduced genetic variation (reflected in a small effective population size) are **population bottlenecks** and **founder effects** (Figure 3.7 and Box 3.2). A population bottleneck occurs when a previously larger population is reduced in number by some event; for example, disease or famine. Even if the population size recovers, the survivors will have only a small proportion of the genetic diversity present in the original population. In a similar way, a founder effect occurs when a small part of a larger population becomes genetically isolated, perhaps by migration or by some geographical event such as rising sea level. The isolated subpopulation will contain only a fraction of the diversity present in the main population. However, studies that attempt to draw conclusions about historical population processes (such as bottlenecks) from the extent of genetic diversity must account for the changes wrought by selection.

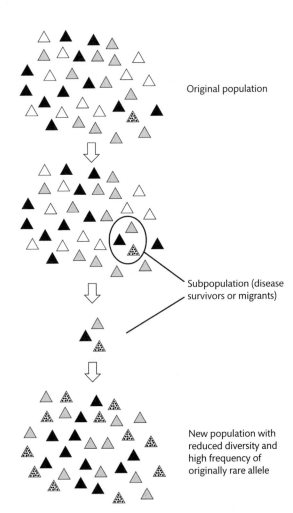

Original population

Subpopulation (disease survivors or migrants)

New population with reduced diversity and high frequency of originally rare allele

Figure 3.7 Bottlenecks and founder effects. A reduction in effective population size, whether because of reduction in total population size by, for example, disease (a bottleneck) or because of isolation of a subpopulation (founder effect), will reduce genetic diversity. Subsequent population expansion is derived from only a small sample of the genetic diversity present in the original population.

Box 3.2 Examples of bottlenecks and founder effects

Founder effects and population bottlenecks have long-term effects on populations. The mapping of many rare diseases that are prevalent in the Finnish population and the homogeneity of Native American blood types are examples.

The Finnish population is a highly isolated population formed approximately 2000 years ago by a founder population characterized by low population count, homogeneity, and isolation. The Eastern Finnish population is estimated to have been founded by only 20–30 families. Thus, although a rapid population increase occurred, the Finns remained a highly homogeneous community. As geneticists began to use technology to map diseases, the Finns became a source of intense interest when more than 33 rare genetic diseases were found to be more prevalent in the Finnish population than in other populations. The term 'Finnish disease heritage' was coined to refer to these oddly prevalent genetic disorders. Congenital nephrosis was one of the first of these rare diseases found to

occur in the Finnish population. Another example is aspartylglucosaminuria, which occurs when lysosomal aspartylglucosaminidase activity is deficient, causing gradual mental retardation. Although in other populations several different mutations can cause this disease, an identical mutation was found in 98% of cases in Finland, suggesting that almost all the Finnish cases arise from a single founder event. There is no doubt that the prevalence of so many such rare diseases could not occur without the largely isolated, homogenous founder population characteristic of the Finns.

Founder effects and population bottlenecks have caused a high level of homogeneity in Native Americans as well. The effective population size of the founder population of the Americas may have been as few as 100 individuals. One of the most interesting results of this lack of diversity is the homogeneity of blood types. Individuals of Amerindian descent are found to mostly have blood of type O.

3.4.2 Molecular effects of selection

This book is about evolution: selection on inherited variation. How does selection affect diversity, and what can we infer about past selective pressures from studies of current human diversity?

Selection will actively affect allele frequencies by increasing the frequency of advantageous alleles in the population (**positive selection**) and decreasing the frequency of deleterious alleles (**negative selection**). Modelling shows that even weakly advantageous alleles will increase rapidly (in evolutionary terms) in frequency in an ideal (i.e. infinitely large) population; for example, an allele that imparts a 1% advantage in fitness will increase to 50% frequency in a population within a few hundred generations. In humans, changes in allele frequency on that scale would take several thousand years, and indeed this is the timescale observed when we look at human alleles which have undergone recent selection,

such as that for lactase persistence. But the effect on the frequency of the allele is a balance between random drift and selection, with population size again playing a major role in which factor predominates. For example, in a small population beneficial alleles may be eliminated or deleterious alleles may become established by random drift before their frequency can be affected by selection.

Importantly for our later discussion of inherited disease, the selection pressure on an allele may be dependent on whether it is dominant or recessive and whether it is expressed homozygously or heterozygously. Recessive alleles may be invisible to selection unless they are expressed homozygously, which is one of the reasons why deleterious alleles can persist within a population. Rarely, a new allele may be selected because it increases the fitness of heterozygotes relative to either of the homozygotes (i.e. individuals carrying two ancestral alleles or two new alleles), a situation known as a **balancing polymorphism** or **heterozygote advantage**. The best known examples in humans are the various red blood cell disorders associated with protection against malaria infection (see section 3.6).

3.4.3 Signatures of selection

The extent of the molecular changes that contributed to the early evolution of the human lineage can be estimated by comparison of the human DNA sequence with that of our closest recent ancestor, the chimpanzee, and even from comparisons with the fragmentary DNA sequences available from neanderthal DNA (see Chapter 6). But is it possible to identify selection that has occurred more recently, providing evidence for the selective pressures that have acted on modern humans?

Tests for selection generally compare observed patterns of diversity with the patterns predicted by neutral evolution, with the assumption that any difference must be a result of selection. Such tests analyse a large amount of DNA sequence data and are therefore dependent on advanced statistical and computational techniques known as bioinformatics.

One test for selection is to compare the pattern of synonymous and non-synonymous mutations in protein-coding regions. Since synonymous changes have no effect on the sequence of the protein product, they are assumed to reflect neutral evolution, whereas non-synonymous changes are assumed to reflect selection. A drawback of this method is its limitation to the small proportion of protein-coding sequence in the genome, whereas it is becoming increasingly apparent that selection on regulatory and structural regions of the genome also has important evolutionary effects.

A more general method is to study patterns of linkage disequilibrium and haplotype diversity. The principle behind this approach is that an allele strongly favoured by selection will rise rapidly in frequency in the population, bringing with it adjacent regions of the chromosome on which it lies (genetic hitch-hiking). This **selective sweep** results in reduced genetic diversity around the target allele. In practice, this reduced diversity is detected as a long haplotype, because if the selective sweep is recent there will have been little time for the surrounding region to be perturbed by mutation or recombination (Figure 3.8). Such methods have been used to generate maps of recent positive selection in geographically sepa-

rated human populations, revealing both shared and region-specific signals; the genes identified as targets of selection included both expected (for example, lactase persistence, metabolism, and skin pigmentation) and unexpected (for example, drug-metabolizing enzymes) candidates (Table 3.1).

3.5 From genotype to phenotype

So far in this chapter we have discussed the basis of genetic diversity – variations in the genotype. To appreciate how genetic variation may contribute to physical characteristics or to disease, we need to know how changes in the nucleotide sequence of DNA are reflected in the phenotype. It is important to note that most genetic variation does not result in any detectable change in phenotype: the change may not occur in a protein-coding region or may result in a synonymous change that has no effect on the protein product. Even if the variation does cause some change in gene expression, the **robustness** of developmental processes may mean that there is no corresponding change in phenotype (for example due to canalization; see Chapter 4).

If a change in DNA sequence has an effect on an individual's phenotype, then in the majority of cases it is because the change has occurred in a protein-coding or regulatory sequence and the amount or activity of a protein product has been altered. Such changes may be dramatic, such as a complete absence of the functional protein, or more subtle, such as production of a protein with a slight change in its function.

Inherited disease is conventionally divided into two types, as follows.

- There are single-gene or **Mendelian** disorders, where the phenotype is determined by a mutation at an individual locus that is inherited in the simple manner described by Gregor Mendel. Mendelian disorders such as cystic fibrosis are rare.
- There are **multifactorial** disorders, where the phenotype is determined by variations at a few or many different loci. The most common of human disorders such as cardiovascular disease and type 2 diabetes are generally multifactorial, with susceptibility determined by the combined influence

antibiotic regimens, and digestive-enzyme replacement therapy mean that many individuals with cystic fibrosis survive into their fourth or fifth decade.

The gene for CFTR is on chromosome 7q31.2. Over 1000 mutations in this gene have been identified; the most frequent, occurring in 60–80% of cases, is a three-base-pair deletion causing the loss of a phenylalanine residue at position 508 of the protein (Δ-F508); the faulty Δ-F508 protein is destroyed by the cell's quality-control mechanisms before it reaches the cell surface. Cystic fibrosis is a recessive disorder: homozygotes have a complete lack of functional protein whereas heterozygote carriers have one functional copy of the gene and appear phenotypically normal.

Cystic fibrosis is the most common lethal genetic disorders in European populations, with an average prevalence of 1 in 2500, implying an allele frequency of 0.02. However, the disease is much less common in other populations, with allele frequencies of 0.01 in Africa and 0.002 in East Asia. Within Europe, there is a clinal gradient of allele frequency, decreasing from north to south. The age of the Δ-F508 mutation in European populations has been estimated to be at least 600 generations (about 15 000 years).

The early lethality of homozygosity for cystic fibrosis raises the question of why the allele has not been removed from the population by selection. Proposals of a hypothetical heterozygote advantage for cystic fibrosis alleles must provide a plausible molecular basis as well as explain the high prevalence in northern Europe. The first hypothesis involved protection against diarrhoeal disease. Bacteria that cause secretory diarrhoea, such as

Vibrio cholerae and some strains of *Escherichia coli*, produce toxins that interact with the CFTR on the intestinal epithelium. Furthermore, the bacterium that causes typhoid uses wild-type CFTR to enter gastrointestinal epithelial cells, and cells expressing the Δ-F508 variant contain many fewer bacteria. Nevertheless, the European preponderance of cystic fibrosis poses a problem for this model: diarrhoeal disease is common worldwide and if anything shows an opposite gradient to that of cystic fibrosis, being more prevalent in tropical regions. Moreover, it is unlikely that cholera was present in Europe before the early part of the nineteenth century, making it unlikely that cholera infection provided strong selective pressure favouring cystic fibrosis alleles in European populations before that time.

A more recent hypothesis suggests that tuberculosis may be the disease against which cystic fibrosis provides heterozygote advantage. The historical and geographical distribution of cystic fibrosis is more consistent with that of tuberculosis than of diarrhoeal diseases. Several studies have reported a reduced frequency of tuberculosis in cystic fibrosis patients and their parents (who must be heterozygotes). Indeed, reduced arylsulfatase activity in patients with cystic fibrosis may inhibit growth of *Mycobacterium tuberculosis* as it lacks arylsulfatase activity and cannot metabolize sulphate, and this provides a molecular explanation for the phenomenon. Modelling studies have demonstrated that the European tuberculosis epidemic that began in the seventeenth century and continued until the late nineteenth century would have provided sufficient selective pressure to account for the current prevalence of cystic fibrosis.

Other examples of Mendelian diseases for which heterozygote advantage has been postulated include cystic fibrosis and Tay-Sachs disease. Balancing selection may also contribute to diversity in the major histocompatibility complex (MHC) genes (see Chapter 9), where such diversity maximizes the range of epitopes to which the immune system can respond.

Finally, the changing environment of humans alters the background on which selection operates. We can envisage two opposing factors will affect how selection operates on Mendelian disease. First, improvements in medical care mean that individuals with diseases that in the past severely limited fitness are now able to have children, reducing the selective pressure that tended to eliminate the causative alleles from the population. Conversely, improvements in public health to reduce the burden of infectious disease mean a reduction in the power of the forces that have driven balancing selection, decreasing the heterozygote advantage that has maintained deleterious alleles in the population.

3.7 No single genes for common diseases

For the common diseases such as obesity, type 2 diabetes, and cardiovascular disease there is no single causative gene. Rather, susceptibility to such diseases probably arises from the combined effects of numerous risk alleles, each with small effect, coupled with environmental and developmental factors (see Chapters 4 and 8). Moreover, how those risk alleles combine to affect risk of disease is not simple to predict. Interactions may be additive or synergistic (**epistatic**) and may be subject to threshold effects, and gene–environment interactions may affect the penetrance of the alleles.

If certain diseases are common, could the alleles causing them also be common: the 'common disease/common variant' hypothesis? Or could they be caused by multiple, but individually rare, alleles at disease loci? This question has implications for the strategies of searching for such alleles (see Box 3.4, below). In fact, both situations seem to occur. For example, some of the heritable variation in plasma low-density lipoprotein cholesterol levels is caused by multiple rare alleles in the *NPC1L1* gene, whose product mediates intestinal cholesterol transport and is the molecular target of the cholesterol-lowering drug ezetimibe. Conversely, a common variant in the *FTO* gene, for which about 16% people of European origin are homozygous (allele frequency 0.4 by Hardy–Weinberg equilibrium), increases the risk of obesity and therefore of type 2 diabetes. Another common SNP associated with obesity and insulin resistance has recently been found in the control region of the melanocortin-4 receptor (MC4R) gene, which is involved in regulating appetite and energy balance. The effect of the *MC4R* risk allele (allele frequency about 0.25 in northern European populations) is additive to that of the *FTO* risk allele. Interestingly, the *MC4R* risk allele is more common (allele frequency 0.37) in individuals of South Asian descent, who are known to be more susceptible to central adiposity and insulin

resistance. The MC4R polymorphism, which presumably modulates the expression of the receptor protein in some way, is of particular note. Loss-of-function mutations in the coding region for the receptor protein have long been known to be associated with a rare and dominantly inherited syndrome characterized by early-onset hyperphagia and morbid obesity, thus revealing overlap in the genetic causes of monogenic and multifactorial metabolic dysfunction. Whether this will be a recurring pattern remains to be elucidated.

But even for *FTO*, so far the best-characterized gene increasing the risk of obesity and type 2 diabetes, the effects on disease risk are modest and population-specific. For example, in Europeans, homozygosity for the *FTO* risk allele increases adult body mass by only about 3 kg and increases the risk of obesity by 1.67-fold and the risk of metabolic syndrome 1.17-fold compared with individuals who do not carry the risk allele. Yet such allele frequencies and increased risk are not seen in all human populations. Furthermore, even when examined at the level of adipose tissue itself, the contribution of heritability to the expression of obesity-related traits on a genome-wide basis is only of the order of 30%.

Importantly, the effect of risk alleles may be modified by environmental factors. For example, the effects of several genes that increase the risk of type 2 diabetes are modified by birth weight (a proxy for early-life nutrition; see Chapter 7). The peroxisome proliferator-activated receptor γ (PPARγ) Pro-12→Ala/Pro SNP is reported to be associated with a risk of later-life insulin resistance in a Finnish cohort, but only in those of lower birth size. A number of similar interactions have been reported, including an interaction between birth weight, the insulin VNTR locus, and risk of insulin resistance in young adults; and an interaction between birth weight, *ACE* gene polymorphism, and glucose tolerance in the elderly. In the musculoskeletal system there are interactions between birth weight, vitamin D receptor (Figure 3.9) or calcium-sensing receptor genotype, and risk factors for osteoporosis in older adults.

Again, the question arises of why, even if these alleles are only slightly deleterious, they have not been eliminated by selection during human evolutionary history. The reasons are similar to those discussed above for monogenic disorders, but with some nuances. First, slightly deleterious alleles, particularly if common in the population, may not affect fitness to a sufficiently great extent that there is

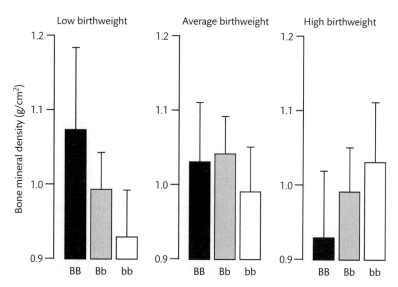

Figure 3.9 Birthweight modifies the relationship between lumbar spine bone mineral density and vitamin D receptor genotype in elderly men and women. Among individuals in the lowest third of birthweight, bone mineral density was significantly higher among individuals of genotype BB. In contrast, bone mineral density was reduced in individuals of the same genotype who were in the highest third of birthweight (from Gluckman, P.D. *et al.* (2008) *New England Journal of Medicine* **359**, 61–73, with permission).

strong selection pressure against them, especially if they are only deleterious in combination with other alleles. And, of course, effects which appear after reproductive age, as is generally the case with most of these chronic diseases, will affect fitness even less. Second, alleles that once were advantageous or neutral in the environments in which humans evolved may now be deleterious in the very different environments in which most of us now live. Thus, it is the interaction with evolutionarily novel environments (for example, increased lifespan or energy-rich nutrition) that causes genetic variation expressed in the phenotype to manifest as ill-health. Applied specifically to energy metabolism, this is the basis of the **thrifty genotype hypothesis** discussed further in Chapter 8.

Furthermore, such now-deleterious alleles may be the targets of selection in current human populations, but because of the slow pace of selection they will still be common. There is evidence that selection has operated on some of these susceptibility genes for common diseases. For example, the allele of the PPARγ gene which increases susceptibility to type 2 diabetes is the ancestral allele – the one found in our nearest relative the chimpanzee – whereas the protective allele is human-

specific. Similarly, the risk allele for cardiovascular and Alzheimer's disease of the apolipoprotein E gene (E4) may be the ancestral allele, since it may have a 'thrifty' role in lipid metabolism and also protect against childhood diarrhoea. Recent work has revealed that different human populations apparently show climate-related adaptation in genes associated with some of the common metabolic disorders, suggesting that metabolic function may be subject to the same clinal variation as skin colour and body shape (see Chapter 6) and such variation may underpin population differences in disease susceptibility.

3.8 Non-genetic inheritance

Does genetic variation underlie all transmissible characteristics? Suggestions that transmission across generations can occur by means other than through inheritance of DNA sequence have always been regarded with suspicion by biologists, and referred to pejoratively as 'Lamarckian' (see Chapter 2). Yet there are several other ways in which culture, behaviour, or even physical characteristics can aggregate within families.

Box 3.4 Looking for the genetic causes of complex disease: linkage versus association

There are two broad approaches to finding genes associated with inherited disease. The first is **linkage mapping**, which attempts to find correlations between patterns of disease occurrence in families and patterns of transmission of genetic markers, such as known genes with obvious phenotypic effects, or particular DNA sequences. If disease susceptibility is transmitted in the same pattern as the marker, then the disease-causing gene must be physically close to the marker (because they are not being separated by recombination). Knowledge of the genes present on the chromosome region identified by the marker furnishes a list of **candidate genes** whose contribution to disease causation can be examined by molecular biological methods and by assessment of biological plausibility. Linkage mapping is most effective for highly penetrant monogenic disorders. There are many sampling and statistical issues in analysing patterns of multilocus genetic variation. Consequently, many early linkage studies that claimed to identify genes involved in complex multifactorial disorders have not been replicated.

The second approach comprises **association studies**, which analyse unrelated people with and without a disease (cases and controls, respectively) for the presence of particular alleles. If an allele is found more often in cases than in controls, then it (or a closely linked allele) is assumed to play a role in the disease. The availability in the last few years of large data sets of human genetic variation and of array technology allowing simultaneous analysis of hundreds of thousands of SNPs, together with assembly of large cohorts (thousands or tens of thousands of individuals) of cases and controls, has paved the way for **genome-wide association studies** that have identified genetic variation contributing to several multifactorial diseases. For example, a recent study of 14 000 cases of seven common diseases and 3000 shared controls identified disease loci for coronary heart disease, type 1 and type 2 diabetes, rheumatoid arthritis, Crohn's disease, bipolar disorder, and hypertension. Again, conclusions drawn in one study alone must be interpreted with caution: replicability may be limited for the same statistical and technical reasons discussed above. It is also important to remember that these are simply association studies and do not demonstrate cause and effect: the presence of an allele does not necessarily or directly confer a risk of the disease. The association may be indirect, the allele may be a contingent factor dependent on the presence of other factors, genetic, developmental, or environmental. Thus there are many reasons both technical and biological for why associations in one population are not necessarily seen in another.

The first is cultural inheritance, where people learn ways of thinking and acting from other people. Cultural inheritance does not simply involve children learning from their parents: individuals may learn from other members of their parents' generation or from their peers. The behaviours acquired may be both positive (for example, attitudes to education or career opportunities) or negative (for example, copying of damaging patterns of eating, smoking, or drug abuse) for health, and it is easy to see how, for example, obesity may aggregate in families because of transmission of attitudes to exercise and eating patterns between generations. Indeed, a recent study indicates that obesity may be 'transmissible' within social networks within the same generation, with increased risk of a person becoming obese if a sibling, friend, or spouse themselves became obese.

Behaviour may also be transmitted without requiring active learning. Rat mothers differ in the amount of attention they pay to their pups, with some mothers licking and grooming their pups often and other mothers doing so

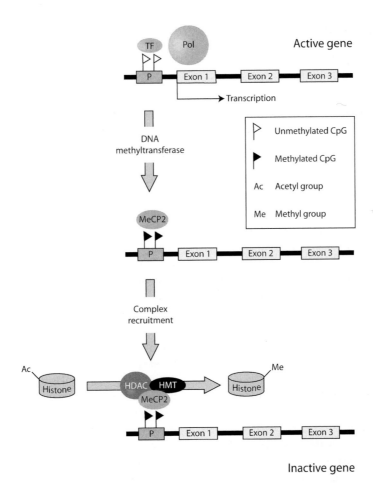

Figure 4.5 Epigenetic modulation of gene expression. When CpG dinucleotides in the gene promoter (P) are unmethylated, transcription factors (TF) and RNA polymerase (Pol) can bind to their specific nucleotide sequences and transcription of coding sequences (Exons) occurs. Methylation of CpGs by DNA methyltransferases causes binding of methyl-CpG binding protein-2 (MeCP2), which in turn recruits the histone-modifying enzymes histone deacetylase (HDAC) and histone methyltransferase (HMT) to form a complex bound to the promoter. The MeCP2-HDAC-HMT complex removes acetyl groups from histones and catalyses methylation of specific lysine residues. This causes the chromatin strand to adopt a 'tighter' conformation, preventing access of transcription factors and RNA polymerase to the DNA and resulting in silencing of transcription (previously published in Gluckman, P.D. *et al.* (2009) *Nature Reviews Endocrinology* volume 5).

DNA methylation also plays a key role in cell differentiation by silencing the expression of specific genes during the development and differentiation of individual tissues. This is the basis of cell differentiation, and pluripotent stem cells retain the ability to make epigenetic changes at the appropriate time. The difference between two cell types from the same individual lies in the epigenetic profile determining which genes are functional and under what conditions. For example, the expression of the homeobox (Hox) gene *Oct-4*, a key regulator of cellular pluripotency in the early embryo, is permanently silenced by hyper-methylation of its promoter around embryonic day 6.5 in the mouse, while *HoxA5* and *HoxB5*, which are required for later stages of development, are not methylated and silenced until early postnatal life. For some genes there also appear to be gradations of promoter demethylation associated with developmental changes in the role of the gene product. The δ-crystallin II and PEPCK promoters are methylated in the early embryo, but undergo progressive demethylation during fetal development and are fully demethylated and expressed in the adult. Thus functional changes in different cell lineages are established at different times during development of the embryo. The established pattern of DNA methylation is then copied during mitosis by DNA methyltransferase 1 activity. This provides an 'epigenetic memory' of patterns of gene regulation, and hence cell type and function, which once established during development is passed through subsequent cell divisions. This discussion has focused on cell differentiation but the same processes can inform the function of regulatory systems in these cells. This immediately suggests a mechanism by which the environment may induce stable changes to cell function which persist into adulthood, and therefore by which environmental challenges at different times during development may produce different phenotypic outcomes, and so differential risk of disease.

Genomic imprinting (see Chapter 7), in which the expression of an allele depends on its parent of origin, represents a special case of epigenetic regulation of gene expression (genomic imprinting should not be confused with the behavioural imprinting studied by Konrad Lorenz, most famously with his geese). Imprinting is most frequently mediated by allele-specific DNA methylation, although imprinted alleles may differ in other ways. Beckwith–Weidemann syndrome results from biallelic expression of insulin-like growth factor 2 (IGF-2) whereas under normal conditions only the paternal allele is expressed. The result is a neonate who is abnormally large with hyperinsulinaemia. This leads to hypoglycaemia and thus a risk of brain damage; these individuals also have an increased risk of developing cancers. Although there are several ways in which Prader–Willi and Angelman syndromes can arise, both involve the same locus on chromosome 15q encompassing several imprinted genes. Prader–Willi syndrome is the result of loss of the active paternal allele (the maternal allele normally being silenced) and Angelman syndrome is the loss of the maternal allele (because there is one gene at the locus which is normally silenced on the paternally inherited chromosome). The phenotypes that arise are quite different: Prader–Willi syndrome is characterized by obesity and hyperphagia, mild mental retardation, hypotonia, and hypogonadism, whereas Angelman syndrome shows developmental delay, hand-flapping, seizures, and a happy demeanour. Although rare, the incidence of imprinting disorders and particularly Beckwith–Weidemann syndrome is apparently increased in offspring conceived by assisted reproductive techniques. However, there is now a report that the risk of other conditions such as cardiovascular disease and type 2 diabetes is also increased in people conceived by in vitro fertilization, and a component of these conditions is thought to involve non-imprinted genes (see below).

Epigenetic mechanisms allow another level of control on top of the genetic code itself. Three aspects of the process are of interest in the current context. The first is that epigenetic changes usually do not involve the coding regions of the genes themselves; rather they affect the gene promoters and genomic regions well upstream. This means that they do not affect gene transcription until the appropriate transcription factor is present. This allows for the phenotype to be affected in a contingent way, as it will alter the future responses of the individual to an environmental challenge which changes levels of the relevant transcription factors. The second aspect is related: namely, it provides an explanation for how a challenge during development, which did not overtly disrupt that development, can have distant effects at a later stage in the life course. The third perspective arising from these epigenetic concepts is that they stand distinct from genetic determinism. They offer ways in which interventions could potentially reverse epigenetic changes set up in early life, if they can be identified and rectified within the critical window of plasticity. This will be challenging but not impossible (laboratory methods to assess DNA methylation and histone modification are available, and pharmacological and nutritional manipulation of epigenetic state is being tested experimentally). Epigenetic change has also been implicated in some cancers, and may provide a therapeutic target; histone deacetylase inhibitors have already entered clinical trials in oncology.

4.7 Intergenerational effects

Most epigenetic marks are erased during gametogenesis and embryogenesis. It was once thought that they were *all* erased, but it is now clear this is not the case, providing the potential for a non-genomic form of biological inheritance. There are human examples of disease risk related to environment being passed across several generations; for example, the relation between risk of adult diabetes in men and the nutritional environment of their grandfathers before puberty, or the higher adiposity in grandchildren of people exposed to famine in the Western Netherlands at the end of the Second World War. There

Box 4.4   Epigenetic marking in human twins

Are the epigenetic 'marks' on the genome which are established during development permanent? They are usually thought to be so in most cells, although the pathological changes occurring in cancer are associated with disordered epigenetic control of processes such as the cell cycle. But one way of examining this concept is to examine epigenetic patterns in identical twins, who have identical genomic DNA. Fraga and his colleagues showed that in fact the patterns of global DNA methylation of these twins are not identical, and that they become more disparate as they get older. Figure 4.6a shows the stark difference in global DNA methylation in 3-year-old and 50-year-old monozygous twin pairs.

The dramatic increase in DNA methylation with age in turn translates to a 4-fold difference in number of differentially expressed genes of younger and older twin pairs (Figure 4.6b). This is a vivid illustration of how different phenotypes can arise from the same genotype, and the contribution of epigenetic modification to the process.

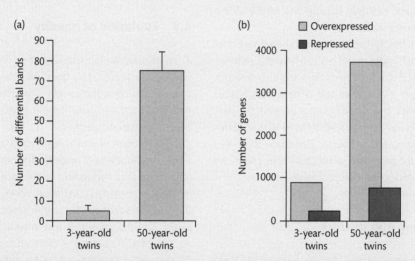

Figure 4.6 Epigenetic differences in twins increase with age. The figure shows the number of differentially methylated regions in a sample of genomic sequences (left panel) and the estimated total number of differences in gene expression (right panel) in monozygotic twins of different ages (modified from Fraga, M. *et al.* (2005) *Proceedings of the National Academy of Sciences USA* **102**, 10604–10609, with permission).

are some experimental data showing that phenotypic characteristics such as blood pressure, heart dimensions, metabolism and HPA axis settings of animals can be altered by endocrine or nutritional manipulations of their grandmothers, without further environmental challenges to the intermediate generation (their mothers).

The mechanisms of molecular epigenetic inheritance remain poorly understood. Three forms of epigenetic inheritance have been suggested. First, epigenetic marks clearly are maintained through mitosis, and there is some limited evidence they can be maintained through meiosis. Micro-RNAs are present in both sperm and ova and these may be the mode of mark transmission allowing methylation and histone changes to be re-established in the next generation. There is more uncertainty as to whether methylation marks *per se* can pass meiosis. Second, an indirect form of epigenetic inheritance is also possible, where the developmental niche inducing the epigenetic change is re-created in each generation. For example, the size of the uterus is related to a woman's early growth, and so a small mother will grow to have a smaller uterus. She will in turn support a smaller baby who thus develops an altered epigenetic profile and grows to have a smaller uterus, and so on. Third, the female gametes (ova) are all formed in the human female when her ovaries develop while she is still a fetus. Thus, a nutritional challenge to a woman during pregnancy cannot only affect the developmental plasticity of her fetus, but also potentially produce epigenetic effects in her fetus's own ova which will contribute directly to the epigenome of her grandchildren, effectively conferring two generations of epigenetic inheritance but only through the female in the intermediate generation.

The opportunities for such transgenerational transmission seem more limited in the male, where the gametes are formed continuously. Nonetheless, the diabetes data referred to above give an example of how transmission could occur from the grandpaternal generation, perhaps involving small non-coding RNAs in sperm. Male-line effects passing to the fourth generation have also been reported for some environmentally toxic chemicals which have an endocrine disruptor function.

4.8   Learning and instinct

Learning is a particular and distinct form of plasticity which is intimately connected with the more structural (e.g. synaptogenic) and molecular epigenetic processes we have examined. Learning is generally transmitted by instruction or observation between individuals but some behaviours appear to be 'instinctive' rather than learned. The transmission of learned behaviour was considered independently by several theorists at the end of the nineteenth century – Morgan, Osborne, and later Baldwin – and perhaps unjustly has become known as the **Baldwin effect**. In essence, the Baldwin effect proposes an evolutionary mechanism for how a learned behaviour can become innate or instinctive. Once a particularly advantageous behaviour (for example, predator avoidance or a new way to exploit a food source) has been 'discovered', individuals who have improved capacity to learn

that skill will be selected until the behaviour becomes an integral part of the species' genetic repertoire. This is thus another example of genetic assimilation (see Box 4.3). In this way, behaviour can shape the course of evolution of a species.

The Baldwin effect concept is still controversial: there is debate about the extent to which a learned behaviour can eventually be assimilated into the genome and about whether selection can act on specific components of behaviour or just on general learning abilities. In addition it has been argued that the change from learning to genetically determined behaviour (instinct) will not necessarily give greater fitness except in very stable environments where change is extremely slow.

4.9   Evolution of novelty

A major question in macroevolution is how phenotypic novelty is achieved. This question is largely beyond the scope of this book and we will only summarize the issues here because they highlight the importance of adopting a developmental perspective.

The evolution of a phenotypically novel feature, such as the development of limbs in the shift from an aquatic to a terrestrial vertebrate, is dependent on selection acting on phenotypic variation which is underpinned by genomic variation. But any selected variant must be viable, and this generates bias in what can be selected. As an adult phenotype is dependent on the successful and viable development of the organism, studies of how macroevolution occurs have increasingly focused on embryological development and the science of developmental biology. Random mutation has generally been seen as the powerhouse of the generation of novelty, but there may also be other factors at play which facilitate the appearance of new forms. Indeed, most random mutations will be either covert and neutral (unless the environment changes to favour the changed phenotype) or, if they involve a coding region, they may well be lethal. Mutations affecting transcriptional regulation are less likely to be lethal as they will affect the place, magnitude, or timing of the expression of a gene and are more likely to result in viable modification of structure or function.

The early embryo differentiates into a number of compartments because of the expression of diffusible factors

Box 4.5   Multicellularity and complexity

Metazoans are characterized by multicellularity, with their component cells differentiated into specialized types. Differentiated multicellularity was the solution to the problem of increasing body size where unicellular organisms aggregated into colonies: it overcomes constraints on diffusion through the development of specialized functions (e.g. the circulatory system). It provides selective advantage by, for example, a digestive system which secretes enzymes permits digestion of a larger potential food source. Tissue differentiation in turn depends on the evolution of epigenetic mechanisms to regulate tissue-specific gene regulation, and the earliest metazoans such as *Volvox* (a green alga) simply consist of two cell types – nutritional and reproductive – allowing reproduction to occur in some cells while nutritional support is provided by others. In general, the larger an organism, the more complex the organization that is needed.

called morphogens which give it polarity, laterality, and its dorsal-ventral dimensions. In turn, this allows the embryo to start to differentiate. A key feature of embryonic development is the distinct pattern of 'segmentation' both dorso-ventrally and rostro-caudally, and this gives each phylum its distinct organizational characteristics. During development, clusters of genes are activated in strict sequence, determining the overall body pattern in terms of numbers of segments and the orientation of each particular segment, and then sub-clusters of genes specify localized structures such as the particular arrangement of organs and tissues within each segment.

Critical to specifying this body plan are two classes of genes: the segmentation genes, which determine how body segments are divided, and the *Hox* genes, which determine how each individual segment develops. The homeobox is a DNA-binding element in a protein which attaches to promoter regions of other genes and activates them. *Hox* genes therefore code for protein transcription factors which, often working in combination, switch on cascades of gene expression that specify the proteins, and hence the structures, that will be produced in the various segments of the developing embryo. Early work on *Hox* genes was performed in *Drosophila*, which is easy to study because of its rapid life cycle and well-defined adult segments, but very similar *Hox* genes are also present in the genomes of mammals. The *Hox* genes in flies are colinear: arranged on a single chromosome in the order of the body parts which they specify. Although the

genes have been duplicated in mammals to form clusters on four chromosomes, their basic arrangement within each cluster is the same (Figure 4.7).

Segmentation or compartmentalization allows a limited number of genes to serve different functions by being linked together in modules which may evolve functionally for different purposes. Hence fins, wings, and limbs all involve homologous genes in comparable segments evolving differently in different organisms. At one level these modules create a fundamental robustness for the phylum; at another level mutational variation within a module can allow phenotypic change that is more likely to be viable. Mutations of the pattern-forming genes can cause large – but often viable – morphological changes. For example, much early work on *Drosophila* pattern-forming genes was carried out on a mutant with an extra pair of wings in place of stubby structures called balancing organs (halteres). The co-linearity of the relevant genes meant that when the gene which would normally have specified the balancing organ was mutated, the next gene in the sequence came into action and specified a pair of wings instead.

There is a growing body of knowledge that such processes are fundamental components of macroevolution. But equally they can explain certain birth defects in humans. For example the homologue of *Pax6* is involved in eye formation in invertebrates and *Pax6* mutations in humans can cause aniridia, which manifests as alterations in the structure and function of the eye. Mutation

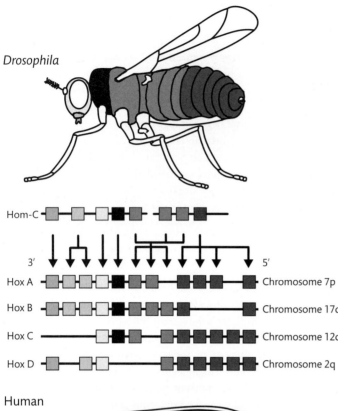

Drosophila

Human

Figure 4.7 Conservation of pattern-forming genes in *Drosophila* and humans. The homeotic (*Hom*) genes in *Drosophila* have duplicated to form the *Hox* gene clusters in vertebrates, but their expression still defines the identities of the same regions of the body (modified from Grier, D.G. *et al.* (2005) *Journal of Pathology* **205**, 154–171, with permission).

of the human homologue of the *Drosophila* segmentation gene *patched* causes the genetic disorder basal cell naevus syndrome, which is characterized by multiple and proliferating skin cancers. Early nutritional deficiencies in the embryo may affect the expression or action of pattern-forming genes, possibly explaining, for example, the gross neural tube defects and anencephaly caused by folate deficiency before neural tube closure is complete.

4.10 Conclusion

Development and its contribution to adaptive processes, and the ways in which the environment affects it, were more or less written out of scientific thought during the twentieth century. But we now realize that even if we succeeded in identifying all the genes which influence a complex trait (see Chapter 3), we would still not be able to describe or predict the expression of that trait in any

---

Box 4.6   The origin of variation

Until around 30 years ago, the conventional explanation for the source of genetic novelties in evolutionary change was mutations in genes coding for the proteins of the altered structure. Then a number of researchers in the emerging field of evolutionary developmental biology began to present a new source of evolutionary mutations: regulatory genes. They maintained that regulatory DNA, known as *cis* elements, had a profound effect on morphological and body-plan changes, and that mutations in this DNA could cause large changes in morphology. For example, in the freshwater and marine varieties of the stickleback fish, the marine species maintain their pelvic skeleton, which serves as a sort of armour, whereas some freshwater species have evolved the total or partial loss of their skeletal armour. The relevant *Pitx* gene was found to be expressed in the pelvic region of the marine species but not the freshwater species, although the sequence of the gene itself remained the same in both groups. This too seems to be evidence that mutations in regulatory *cis*-element DNA, not coding genes that would actually alter the *Pitx* gene sequence, were responsible for these new adaptations.

The role of *cis* elements is a subject of debate, with some investigators maintaining that *cis*-regulatory mutations are significant but do not represent the foundation of morphological evolution. They point to the many more well-documented examples of novelties arising from coding gene mutations, and point out that few of the examples of *cis*-regulatory mutations causing morphological change involve clearly adaptive traits.

---

given individual. This is just as true of disease. It is the triad of *genes*, *development*, and *environment* which is responsible for the adult phenotype of an individual organism, and therefore their susceptibility to disease. The consequences of thinking about the phenotype in this context, rather than focusing on the environment or the genotype alone, should be apparent.

Somatically acquired characteristics cannot be inherited, but environmental influences in one generation can influence subsequent generations through the processes of developmental plasticity and direct or indirect epigenetic inheritance. Modern ideas about non-genomic inheritance, whether mediated by cultural influences, epigenetic changes, or effects on the developmental environment, do not support Lamarck's concept itself, but they nonetheless endorse the idea that phenotype is influenced to a significant degree by these processes, not just by Mendelian genetic inheritance.

Molecular developmental biology has given us many clues about the processes which mediate such effects, especially epigenetic processes. Measurement of epigenetic marks such as DNA methylation in early life now offers the possibility of early diagnosis of disease risk resulting from inappropriate developmental influences, and also of novel interventions and therapies. This area of medicine is the subject of much current research, and clinical application will be realized in the near future.

The challenge for biomedical science is to marry the concepts of evolutionary genetics, developmental biology, and environmental science into a unified vision of what makes us what we are, and how to address the challenges which we face as a species.

KEY POINTS

- The triad of genes, development, and environment is responsible for the adult phenotype of an individual organism.

- Developmental plasticity is the capacity to adjust the phenotype arising from a single genotype by changing pathways of development in early life. It allows organisms to maintain or enhance fitness by matching themselves better to different environments, and to adjust to changing circumstances on a timescale intermediate between that of selection and homeostasis.

- The modularity of structure and function allows for duplication and this can provide an important source of evolutionary novelty.

- Epigenetic molecular processes are central to the mechanisms of developmental plasticity.

- Developmental plasticity, which has an adaptive origin, must be distinguished from developmental disruption, which does not. However, some developmentally plastic responses, while being adaptive in origin, can lead to maladaptive outcomes and may result in impaired health later.

- Environmental influences in one generation can influence subsequent generations through these processes.

Further reading

Gilbert, S.F. (2006) *Developmental Biology*. Sinauer Associates, Sunderland, MA.

Goldberg, A.D., Allis, C.D., and Bernstein, E. (2007) Epigenetics: a landscape takes shape. *Cell* **128**, 635–638.

Gluckman, P.D. and Hanson, M.A. (2005) *The Fetal Matrix: Evolution, Development, and Disease.* Cambridge University Press, Cambridge.

Gluckman, P.D., Hanson, M.A., and Beedle, A.S. (2007) Non-genomic transgenerational inheritance of disease risk. *Bioessays* **29**, 149–154.

Gottlieb, G. (2002) *Individual Development and Evolution: the Genesis of Novel Behavior.* Lawrence Erlbaum Associates, Mahwah, NJ.

Jablonka, E. and Lamb, M.J. (2005) *Evolution in Four Dimensions: Genetic, Epigenetic, Behavioral and Symbolic Variation in the History of Life.* MIT Press/Bradford, Cambridge, MA and London.

Kirschner, M.W. and Gerhart, J. (2005) *The Plausibility of Life: Resolving Darwin's Dilemma.* Yale University Press, New Haven, CT.

Pigliucci, M. and Kaplan, J. (2006) *Making Sense of Evolution: the Conceptual Foundations of Evolutionary Biology.* University of Chicago Press, Chicago, IL.

Schmalhausen, I.I. (1986) *Factors of Evolution: the Theory of Stabilizing Selection.* University of Chicago Press, Chicago, IL.

Waddington, C.H. (1957) *The Strategy of the Genes: a Discussion of Some Aspects of Theoretical Biology.* George Allen & Unwin, London.

West-Eberhard, M.J. (2003) *Developmental Plasticity and Evolution.* Oxford University Press, New York.

Wolpert, L., Beddington, R., Jessell, T. *et al.* (2002) *Principles of Development.* Oxford University Press, Oxford.

CHAPTER 5

Evolution of life histories

5.1 Introduction

Every species has one or more stereotypical patterns that describe its life cycle, and the term **life history** is used to describe this constellation of key characteristics, including the patterns of growth, development, reproduction, and mortality, which define progress through life. Some elements of the life history are common to both male and female, others are gender-specific. Some organisms have alternative life history strategies, called polyphenisms (see Chapter 4), which depend on the environmental cues they received during early development.

There is an enormous diversity in life history strategies across the animal kingdom, but there are also unifying patterns and similarities. Mice are not only much smaller than dogs, humans, or whales, but they also have shorter lifespans. Naturally, their offspring are born much smaller and, perhaps partly as a result, they also have much higher mortality from dangers which large size protects against, such as dying at the hands – or talons – of a predator. Given the higher likelihood that a newborn mouse will end up as a meal for a predator, it would be too risky for the mouse to give birth to a single offspring and instead they give birth to large litters at frequent intervals in the expectation that a few will survive to adulthood to reproduce. Contrast this with the life strategy of an elephant or a human and we begin to see how the characteristics of a species should be envisioned as encompassing much more than just its adult form. Instead, an organism should be viewed as having a strategy of growth, reproduction, and longevity which has been adaptively shaped by natural selection. Life history theory is an important sub-field within evolutionary biology, and its application

provides a valuable window into understanding important aspects of human biology.

Such a comparative approach is a powerful tool, revealing regularities linking traits across the animal kingdom. Defining these relationships is valuable for two reasons. First, it allows the identification of *general patterns* hinting at deeper constraints or underlying processes. Such regularities might, for instance, reflect the limitations of the mechanical properties of bone, the finite energy available for distribution and use within a body of a given size (see below), or something as simple as the need for larger-bodied species to take longer to reach that larger size. Second, it allows us to identify *deviations* from the normal trend, which highlight those instances when selection has pushed a species into an unusual state for that trait. This is illustrated by the example of brain size (see Box 5.4, below).

Understanding both how humans fit within the general mammalian pattern, and those instances in which we deviate from it, has been essential to understanding the evolution of the human life course. Like other selected traits, life history traits are also subject to variation. But within this potential variation there are interactions or trade-offs which constrain the possible life course strategies. For example, across species (and often within a species), there is commonly an association between an earlier age at sexual maturation and a reduced adult body size, and maturation tends to be accelerated when there is a high threat of predation or death. This relationship results because the potential advantage of a larger body size in later life is 'traded-off' against the greater cumulative risk of death from disease or predation during a longer period of maturation. Understanding such trade-offs between life history traits is essential to interpreting many biological strategies. We will return to these themes of shared pattern and uniqueness throughout this chapter.

The human life history is typified by an individual being born to a singleton pregnancy after a gestation of approximately 280 days. This is followed by a long phase of postnatal nutritional dependence on the mother and a prolonged childhood with sexual maturity delayed until more than a decade after birth. Females generally enter puberty before males and there is only modest sexual dimorphism in adult body size. Each female has only a few children and there is high parental investment in each child such that there is a comparatively high probability that children will live to be able to reproduce. Family structures generally involve some form of pair bond between a male and female(s). But whereas males are capable of reproduction into old age, females experience menopause and terminate reproduction before the end of their intrinsic lifespan. The slow intrinsic rate of senescence means that lifespans in excess of 70 years are not exceptional and become the norm when extrinsic causes of death are reduced.

5.2 General overview of life history theory

Assembling data points across a wide array of mammalian species illustrates the range of variation but also the similarities in the linkage between traits such as growth rate, body size, and lifespan. These patterns in turn beg deeper questions about the biological processes which underpin them. What are the differences in biological strategy which distinguish a mouse from a human or an elephant?

Life history theory holds as a central tenet that organisms vary, in large part, because of differences in the ways that they harness and use the finite energy and nutritional resources at their disposal. Functions such as growth, reproduction, and the repair processes that slow ageing and extend lifespan each require energy and commitment of resources. There are constraints on the size of the pool of resources that a species has available to it, and this unavoidably leads to trade-offs between functions. This concept of finite resources provides important

insights into how physiological processes have evolved to balance the trade-offs that necessarily ensue. Before exploring these trade-offs, let us first look at the forces which limit resources.

That an organism must have some upper limit to its energy use is intuitive and has long been appreciated among biologists. Resting metabolic rate can be described as a power function of mass in mammals (Figure 5.1); this is sometimes termed Kleiber's law. Not surprisingly, as one moves from small to large organisms, total energy expenditure increases. What is notable, however, is that energy expenditure increases at a rate *slower* than the increase in body mass. As a result, an elephant may expend more joules per hour in total than a mouse, but a kilogram of elephant requires less energy than a kilogram of mouse. Larger organisms tend to be more efficient than smaller ones. As can be seen in the figure, this relationship is quite regular, with metabolic rate scaling to body mass as a power function with an exponent of 0.75.

This mathematical relationship linking metabolic rate with size reveals that there are limits to the energy available for use within a body of a given mass. Between-species variation in traits such as growth rate, body size, and lifespan results in part from different strategies of energy partitioning (Figure 5.2). Although there is much leeway in the types of allocation strategies which an organism can evolve, it is important to keep in mind the fundamental law of physics that energy must be conserved: a molecule of ATP used in one cell to service one function cannot be used again elsewhere. The simple fact that the pool of resources at any point in an organism's life is finite, and can only be used once, has profound implications for understanding the forces that have shaped the evolution of life history variation. It is also central to understanding how members of a species adapt to environmental challenges such as energetic limitations. Because the body faces trade-offs when allocating resources, species evolved to balance those trade-offs in a fashion that optimizes fitness.

5.2.1 Key trade-offs in life histories

Life history traits that species manipulate (another metaphoric term) to achieve optimal fitness include: the number, size, and sex ratio of offspring; size and maturity at

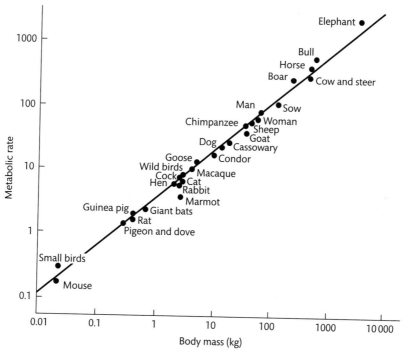

Figure 5.1 The Kleiber line showing scaling of basal metabolic rate against body mass in a number of species (from Bonner, J.T. (2006) *Why Size Matters*. Princeton University Press, Princeton, NJ, with permission).

Box 5.1   The power of quarters

Early proposals to explain Kleiber's law pointed to the fact that an organism's surface area, which radiates heat, increases more slowly than does its volume or mass, which produces it. The geometry of that arrangement implies a scaling component of ⅔ or 0.67, close but not close enough to the 0.75 we can see from the empirical data. Newer concepts look to the geometry of the circulatory system for an explanation. Organisms face an important challenge in distributing resources within their bodies. As blood circulates around the body, it must service all cells in the body; an optimal solution to this problem involves a system of branches upon branches upon branches: beginning with the aorta and branching all the way down to very small capillaries. This type of

nested branching network is an example of what is termed fractal geometry. Although the mathematical proof is beyond the scope of our discussion, because of this geometry the distribution of resources will tend to scale to body mass with an exponent of 0.75, or ¾.

Intriguingly, there are many other relationships within life that scale at the power of a quarter. For instance, animal lifespan is proportional to the quarter power of body mass and heart rate varies inversely with quarter power of body mass. Taking out the body-mass component from those relationships implies that all animals will have a similar number of heartbeats during their lifetime, which is roughly true: about a billion. (Humans, of course, with their anomalously long lifespans, have more: 2–3 billion!) At the ecological level, population density of a species scales inversely to the ¾ power of body mass. There are few species of elephant but many species of insects; indeed, the relationship between body size and diversity follows another quarter-power law. The foraging area of human hunter-gatherer bands is proportional to the ¾ power of group size. And finally, returning to the metabolic level, calculation of drug dose according to body mass (for instance, in adapting an adult dose for a child) is often improved by a ¾ power relationship.

birth; pattern of growth; age and size at maturity; parental investment in offspring; and the investment in repair and maintenance affecting intrinsic mortality and lifespan. There is an extraordinary variation in the solutions that different species of mammal have evolved, each providing an adaptive solution to maintaining gene flow within their usual environment(s). Despite this variation, there are trade-offs that constrain the possible solutions, some of which are described in the following sections.

5.2.1.1 Number versus quality of offspring

Some species give birth to many offspring, of which few survive. This strategy is typical of rodent species. Parental investment in these offspring is low, if not non-existent, once weaning has occurred. Other species such as humans and other large mammals give birth to a single offspring and invest heavily to nourish and protect that offspring at least until it reaches the juvenile stage. These examples represent two extremes of a range of potential approaches.

5.2.1.2 Current versus future reproduction

Another reproductive trade-off is between reproducing now and reproducing in the future. At one extreme are species such as the salmon and the males of some species of marsupial, which reproduce once before dying (termed semelparous breeding). These species invest enormous effort in producing a large number of offspring in a single mating event that exhausts their energetic capacity but is a successful fitness strategy for these species. At the other extreme are species that invest in reproduction across multiple reproductive events and have long reproductive lifespans. Human females limit their energetic investment in an individual pregnancy by generally only conceiving a single fetus, but nevertheless that investment is very high given the prolonged gestation and energetic demands of lactation. Female humans have a potential reproductive life of about 15–35 years after puberty, depending on their extrinsic mortality risk. However, over that period of time relatively few children are born and nurtured, and fitness therefore depends on

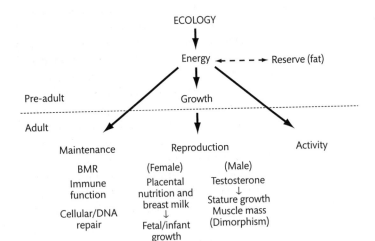

Figure 5.2 Energy allocation to life history traits. BMR, basal metabolic rate (from Kuzawa, C.W. (2007) *American Journal of Human Biology* **19**, 654–661, with permission).

a high proportion (in comparative terms) of these off-spring surviving. Female hunter-gatherers generally have four to six children over their life time with two to four surviving to adulthood.

Females limit their investment in each fetus by mechanisms which restrict nutrient flow to the fetus (a phenomenon termed maternal constraint; see Chapter 7). The first-born child in humans is on average about 150 g lighter than subsequent children. The proximate explanation may be that the uterine arteries cannot dilate as well in the first compared with the subsequent pregnancies, because the elastin in the arterioles and arteries breaks down during the initial pregnancy, leading to a lower vascular resistance (the uterine arteries have to dilate considerably in pregnancy and fetal oxygen delivery is limited by uterine arterial blood flow). But there is also a life history perspective: primates may have evolved with a restriction on energy utilization in the first pregnancy, which has the benefit of conserving energy for subsequent pregnancies.

5.2.1.3 Age versus size at maturity

A defining life history trait is the timing of sexual maturation, and this is discussed in detail in Chapter 7. Depending on the species, growth may stop or slow at or soon after sexual maturity. The trade-off here is between investing energy in continued growth versus investing available energy into reproduction. Models of mammalian life histories generally assume that there are two competing factors which determine the optimal timing of this transition. The first is the importance of adult size to reproductive success. To the extent that body size influences reproductive fitness (by allowing females greater investment in larger, more resilient offspring with lower mortality), this will favour a delay in onset of reproduction. This reproductive benefit must be balanced against a second factor: namely the excess risk of dying, which increases as maturation is delayed. Thus where organisms face a high mortality risk, particularly in the juvenile phase, there is a generally a shorter time to maturation.

5.2.1.4 Fecundity versus lifespan

Fecundity is the measure of the total lifetime reproductive performance of an organism. In female mammals, fecundity is measured by the cumulative number of offspring from a lifetime of multiple pregnancies. But pregnancy and lactation are energetically expensive for the mother and divert resources from maintenance functions. This trade-off is one reason why there is a reciprocal relationship between lifespan and fecundity

---

Box 5.2   A royal trade-off

Does the trade-off between longevity and fecundity operate in humans? To investigate this would require an extensive data set of the lives of individuals under natural fertility (pre-contraception) conditions. Historical reality means that such records have generally only been kept for the wealthy, and indeed one data set used by gerontologists to study this question involves the genealogical records of the British aristocracy, which go back some 1200 years and record information for over 33 000 individuals. As predicted by life history theory, in this population there was a negative correlation between longevity in women and the number of children that they had (the effects of childbirth mortality were accounted for by considering only women who reached their post-reproductive years).

The individuals represented in these records were of course privileged, in that they were presumably insulated from the social and economic contexts of their times. Does the relationship still hold for a 'normal' (socioeconomically heterogeneous) population? A similar analysis of demographic data from northern Germany in the eighteenth and nineteenth centuries found an increasingly strong negative relationship between longevity and fecundity with increasing poverty. This is what would be expected if the trade-off is mediated by resource availability.

across species (short-lived animals tend to have more offspring). Lifespan is by definition shorter where there is a high extrinsic mortality rate, and in species where this occurs one fitness-enhancing strategy is to have high fecundity.

5.2.2 Extrinsic and intrinsic mortality

A key determinant of the life history strategy that a species evolves with is its mortality risk profile. Allocating resources to maintenance functions such as tissue repair can be interpreted in a metaphoric sense as representing an 'expression of optimism', that the organism is likely to live into the future, and thus reap the reproductive rewards of keeping its body functioning and healthy. Thus the rate of unavoidable mortality sets how optimistic and 'forward-looking' a species can afford to be in its life history strategy.

A simple thought experiment illustrates how the optimal life history strategy for a species depends upon the local mortality risk. Imagine a species that inhabits a small island and that faces a source of mortality that is beyond its control, such as lightning strikes. On any given day, there is some small (but not trivial) risk of being struck by lightning. Now, as a result of climate change, the occurrence of lightning increases markedly and the risk of being struck increases dramatically. Note that this ecological change is experienced by each individual organism as a greater risk that, on any given day, it will meet an untimely death. This increase in risk will have several important implications for the species and the life course strategies available to it. The period of growth and development is one in which these risks are greatest from the perspective of fitness optimization. This is not because of the simple fact that the young organism is small and physically vulnerable but rather because from a genetic perspective it has not yet had a chance to reproduce. A juvenile struck by lightning is an individual who will not be represented in the next generation's gene pool. It therefore follows that, as the risk of death on any given day increases, the genes of earlier-reproducing individuals will become more common in the gene pools of subsequent generations. This will lead to a decline in the age of maturity in future generations of offspring.

This evolutionary shift in the age at maturity will have broad and cascading effects on the rest of the species' life history. Assuming that other parameters such as nutrition or growth rate are not affected by the increase in lightning, this reduction in the age at maturity means that there will be less time for growth, and thus, future generations of the adults of this species will also evolve to a smaller final size. This reduction in adult size will, in turn, have additional effects. All else being equal, species that are smaller as adults have less resource to invest in reproduction; that is, in support of fetal and infant growth. Thus, offspring size will also decline as adult size declines. As the size of young decreases, this has additional cascading implications, for it influences how vulnerable each young will be. Small newborns typically have fewer nutritional stores to draw upon, for example for heat generation, in the event of an energy shortfall. They also tend to be more vulnerable to predation. Thus, a by-product of this reduction in offspring size is an increase in offspring mortality. As juvenile mortality increases, it would be too risky for mothers of that species to give birth to a single offspring, for the chances of that offspring making a contribution to the gene pool in the next generation will be very small. As a result, smaller species not only have higher juvenile mortality, but they also tend to 'hedge their bets' by giving birth to litters with multiple offspring. Giving birth to large litters will decrease the size of each offspring further, and thus further increase the risk of fewer offspring reaching adulthood. But this strategy may still yield more surviving offspring than investing in one larger offspring.

Thus we see how a simple change in the local environment – a change in the risk of unavoidable mortality – will tend to have cascading effects on the entire life history. Higher mortality will favour earlier maturation, which will yield smaller adults with fewer metabolic resources and thus a lower capacity to invest in reproduction. This in turn will lead to smaller offspring with higher mortality. As that mortality risk increases, we expect to see an evolutionary shift from singleton births to litters of smaller and more vulnerable offspring.

So far we have seen how a change in local mortality will favour earlier reproductive maturation, and how this in turn will have subsequent effects on adult size, offspring size, offspring mortality, and litter size. These influences are not the only pathway by which a change in mortality will lead to an evolutionary shift in a species' life history. As unavoidable adult mortality increases, investing scarce

10% of the weight of a sparrow or a mouse. Similarly, the shape of trees is affected by their size: larger trees must have thicker stronger trunks as strength is related to the cross-sectional area. Further, the height and shape of trees is affected by competition for sunlight and by the needs of their root systems. Thus the body composition of an organism must change as its size changes. Further the proportions of the body change as an animal grows. Figure 5.9 shows how the relative size of the head changes during growth, being 33% of body length at birth and only 13% in an adult.

Larger objects have a greater surface area, but it does not necessarily increase to the same degree as volume. In a spherical object, surface area is a function of volume$^{2/3}$, and thus complex shapes are needed to have sufficient surface area for diffusion in larger organisms. Placental and intestinal villi, the tortuosity of the gastrointestinal tract, and the alveolar structure of the lungs are all similar solutions to increasing the diffusion area within a constrained space. Similarly, the cortical sulci and gyri of the primate brain are a solution to generating a sufficiently large cortical surface without requiring a gravitationally impossible head.

There are often potential adaptive advantages in having a larger body size, such as providing defence against predators. But there are important constraints including gravity, cardiovascular pump capacity, limb size, diffusion capacity, and nutrient availability. In a stable environment there will inevitably be species of many different sizes, reflecting the multiple ecological niches available. Because there is always a potential niche for a larger organism that can gain advantage through predation of smaller animals or by being more effective at capturing resources (for example by being the highest tree in a forest), there is an impression that over evolutionary time organisms have become larger. But this is not directional evolution, it is simply a reflection of the selective environment and increasing size is not inevitable. In our hypothetical lightning-plagued island, we described how a change in extrinsic mortality may well cause a lineage to evolve to smaller size. 'Island dwarfism' is well described for several mammalian species, including elephants, where a subpopulation has become isolated on a resource-limited island. It has also been evoked as one possible, but controversial, explanation of the recent discovery of skeletal remains of a small hominin on the island of Flores in Indonesia (see Chapter 6).

5.3.1 Allometry

As introduced at the beginning of this chapter, many functions and components of the body are not simply a linear function of body size, and **allometry** is the study of these relationships. For example, the overall weight of an animal is generally a function of the cube of its linear dimensions. However, the strength of bones rises in proportion to the square of their linear dimensions, effectively putting a limit on body size for a land-based animal. The supportive action of water allows animals to grow larger in aquatic environments. These mathematically regular relationships between components of body size and functions across species are known as allometric, and result from generalizable trade-offs between life history traits. A deviation from an expected allometric relationship suggests particular selection for a trait. The most common application of allometric analysis is in the examination of relationships between organ size and body size. A comparative evaluation of brain size in primates and hominins provides an extensive illustration of how allometric analysis can be used (Box 5.4).

5.3.2 Variation in growth and development

There is considerable variation in human size and shape and in the tempo of maturation both within and across

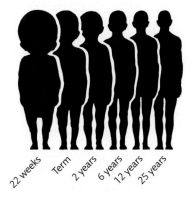

Figure 5.9 Relative head size during human growth (modified from Bonner, J.T. (2006) *Why Size Matters.* Princeton University Press, Princeton, NJ; with permission).

Box 5.4 Brain size

The size and complexity of the human brain allows a sophistication of human social and cultural achievement. We rely upon cognitive ability where other species rely upon traits like brute force, speed, or camouflage. But is the human brain really that special? We think so but how do we go about evaluating this scientifically? As there are limits on assessing functionality in other species, most comparative studies have focused on brain size despite its limitations. Figure 5.10a shows the size of a human brain

relative to other apes, including chimpanzees, gorilla, orang-utan, and the lesser apes, siamangs and gibbons. Also plotted in the same chart is the brain size of a 5000 kg elephant. Looking at raw data is deceptive, because an elephant should have a large brain given their far greater overall body size. And the same is true for the other comparisons, even though the differences in body size are more subtle. What is needed is a comparison of a species' brain size relative to body size. We could simply calculate

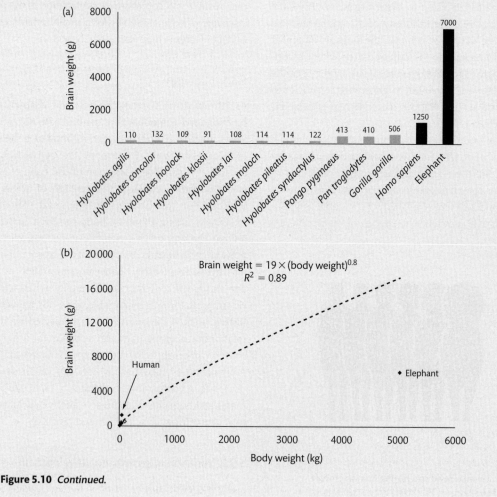

Figure 5.10 *Continued.*

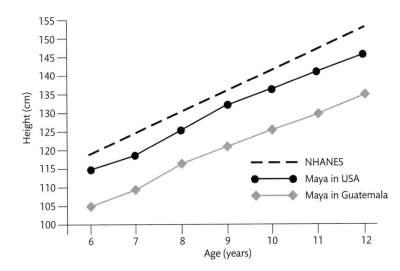

Figure 5.14 Growth curves for Mayan children living in rural Guatemala and for those living in the USA after migration of their parents, compared with US standard growth curves (labelled NHANES). The Mayan children living in the USA are over 10 cm taller than their genetic counterparts living in Guatemala (modified from Smith, P.K. *et al.* (2003) *Economics and Human Biology* **1**, 145–160, with permission).

2–3 years followed by a deceleration which ultimately leads to termination of linear growth with epiphyseal fusion of long bones. The pubertal growth spurt adds about 25 cm in height in females and 27 cm in males. As will be discussed below, the pubertal growth spurt is a unique characteristic of *Homo sapiens*, not seen in other primates: it is thought to have evolved late in the hominin lineage. There are also changes in body proportions as the different components of the skeleton do not all grow synchronously. Thus the span to height ratio changes, with the limbs getting longer relative to the trunk. The relationship of the pubertal growth spurt to reproductive maturation differs between the two genders (Figure 5.15). The initiation of spermatogenesis in males occurs relatively early in puberty at a stage when genital and pubic hair development is only partially progressed and well before peak height velocity is achieved. In contrast, menarche occurs late in the progression of pubertal development in the female, when breast and pubic hair development is almost complete and well after pubertal growth has peaked. There is no event in males equivalent to menarche which allows sexual maturation to be readily assessed; thus most of the discussion will focus on the female, where clearer statements can be made.

Body composition also changes. Whereas females continuously accumulate fat through puberty and adolescence, males have a greater increase in muscle mass and have no overall increase in fat mass (although this is changing as children now have an increased rate of obesity). The possible selective advantage of these different patterns of composition between sexes could be explained in terms of the role of muscle mass in generating fitness in a male (through its potential to affect competition for mates) and of energy stores in doing so in females (i.e. supporting several pregnancies and lactation periods).

The age at onset of puberty varies quite considerably within a population and across populations. The average age at onset of puberty is earlier in the female than in the male. Several factors influence the age at pubertal onset and sexual maturation, including the nutritional state of the girl both *in utero* and in childhood. Some years ago it was suggested that puberty was triggered in girls by a critical percentage of body fat. This so-called Frisch hypothesis did not stand up to critical analysis but it is true that in general better weight gain in childhood is associated with an earlier menarche. The precise mechanisms involved are unclear but the neuroendocrine control of gonadotropin release interconnects with the hypothalamic regulation of satiety and metabolism. Conversely, childhood energy deficits can delay puberty and the onset of menses: this is not uncommonly seen in children who exercise heavily, such as competition gymnasts or ballet dancers, and is a feature of anorexia nervosa. This relationship can

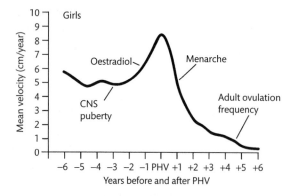

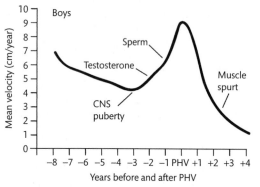

Figure 5.15 Relationship between pubertal growth spurt and timing of events of sexual maturation in girls (top) and boys (bottom). Note that menarche follows peak height velocity (PHV) in girls, whereas sperm production precedes PHV in boys. CNS puberty refers to maturation-related events in the hypothalamus and other brain regions (modified from Bogin, B. (1999) *Patterns of Human Growth*, 2nd edn. Cambridge University Press, Cambridge, with permission).

be interpreted as an override: irrespective of other drivers of maturation, there is an energetic and fitness logic to delaying puberty when nutrients are scarce and energy expenditure levels are high, and permitting an earlier puberty when nutrients are in abundance and require little energy expenditure to obtain. As historically pregnancy generally followed soon after maturation, the variable age of menarche can be interpreted in relation to the energetic costs and fitness effects of a pregnancy at a young age. A pregnancy in conditions of famine is more likely to be associated with a poor outcome and yet to have energetic costs for the mother which may compromise her own survival and future fitness, and thus to

delay maturation in the expectation of potentially better nutritional future is adaptive. Conversely, to be well nourished may allow an earlier puberty, with a longer potential reproductive life and enhanced fitness.

In contrast, *prenatal* growth has the opposite effect. It represents adaptive responses operating over a longer timescale. Children of lower birth weight have accelerated menarche. As discussed in Chapter 7, this has been hypothesized to reflect a shift in developmental trajectory in expectation of living in a more threatening environment. Thus in the phase of developmental plasticity the tempo of development has been shifted in the expectation of a shorter life, and early puberty is an adaptive response to ensure gene flow to the next generation. Those with the earliest puberty are those who are born small and experience greater weight gain in childhood (see Figure 5.6): this is most dramatic in girls adopted from a low-income country into a family in a high-income country.

The initial cycles after menarche are not necessarily associated with ovulation and fertility is not normally maximal until about 2 years after menarche. Further, while the potential mother is young there is a competition between her and her fetus for nutrients as she is still laying down soft tissue for some years after menarche. Thus infants born to young mothers are smaller not only because they are first born but because of nutritional limitations. There may well be an interrelationship between these drivers of smaller birth size and the size of the pelvic inlet. The last component of the skeleton to mature is the pelvic inlet, which generally does not mature until about 17–18 years, and this appears to be independent of the age of menarche. The constraining role of pelvic size in influencing the evolution of the human life history is discussed further in Chapter 7.

5.5 Evolutionary analysis of the distinct features of human growth

When phenotypic change evolves in a lineage it may be that a new structure or control is introduced by way of mutations which lead to a different characteristic; or it may be that during development the timing of the appearance of a feature is altered in relation to others (a process known as **heterochrony**), either because of the bipedal. The evolutionary explanations for bipedalism and its consequences are discussed below. It seems that it preceded the appearance of a larger neocortex. Other novelties which evolved within the hominin clade included a change in dentition and jaw shape and the development of technology and culture.

The early Australopithecine species were bipedal, sexually dimorphic (see Chapter 7), and weighed up to about 45 kg with a brain size of about 400–500 cm^3, giving them a slightly larger brain relative to body size than the modern chimpanzee. They were probably exclusively vegetarian and lived in a woodland habitat. The famous skeleton of Lucy, which is dated about 3 MYA and was discovered by the Leakeys in Olduvai Gorge, is the best-known Australopithecine. An analysis of her skeleton suggests that Lucy was adapted for bipedal walking but was not able to run efficiently. By 2.5 MYA so-called robust Australopithecine species appeared which had greater encephalization. Studies of their teeth suggest they were primarily plant eaters but did include some meat in their diet.

Beginning about 2.5 MYA a further radiation occurred, and species of hominin appeared with smaller jaws and teeth but with a clear increase in brain size. There was probably more meat in the diet although it is not clear whether this was hunted: more likely it was scavenged. Tool use appears for the first time in our ancestral history. This cluster of features marks the appearance of the first species of the genera *Homo*.

These definitions of genera and species are somewhat arbitrary, and there are authorities who lump, and others who split, the scanty evidence to proclaim either fewer or more species. The difficulty is that variation is a characteristic within any species. When relying solely on skeletal data without access to a large number of specimens or to molecular or reproductive behaviour it is not possible to distinguish unequivocally between variation within a species and variation between species.

The earliest member of the genus *Homo* was *Homo habilis*, which had a brain size of more than 600 cm^3 and a body size of about 45 kg, showing greater encephalization. These early species of *Homo* gave rise to a species with a larger body and larger brain, *H. erectus*. The 'Turkana boy' who died about 1.6 MYA is estimated to have been destined for an adult height of 1.85 m and had a cranial capacity of 880 cm^3.

The nomenclature regarding our forebears can be confusing: some authorities refer to the earliest forms of *H. erectus* as *Homo ergaster*, which in turn gave rise to *H. erectus* and *Homo heidelbergenesis*, which in turn is considered the precursor of *H. sapiens* and *Homo neanderthalensis*. The issues surrounding these distinctions are not relevant to this book and so we will use *H. erectus* to include *H. ergaster* and *H. heidelbergenesis*.

Skeletal remains of *H. erectus* have been found not only in Africa but also throughout Indonesia (where the first fossils were found), China, and the Urals. While *H. erectus* evolved about 2 MYA, it migrated out of Africa into Asia only about 1 MYA (although there are some data suggesting an earlier date in the Urals). *H. erectus* appears to have had a prolonged childhood and a life history pattern intermediate between that of modern great apes and humans. This estimate is based on calculations of tooth eruption patterns and of pelvic size to estimate brain size at birth and mature brain size. Hand axes appeared as a new kind of tool, and the archaeological evidence has been interpreted to suggest that *H. erectus* engaged in hunting and had more meat in its diet.

At least two species evolved from *H. erectus*: *H. sapiens* and *H. neanderthalensis*. The latter may have evolved as early as 500 000 years ago and was restricted to Europe and the Middle East. The most recent Neanderthal remains found date to 25 000 to 30 000 years ago. Recently it has been possible to sequence DNA fragments from Neanderthal bones and it is clear they were not a subspecies of *H. sapiens* but a distinct species which could not interbreed with *H. sapiens*. Neanderthals were a highly successful species in the period 100 000–30 000 years ago: they had brains with a volume 10% greater than modern humans. They were more robust with relatively shorter limbs. Their skulls were characterized by sloping brows and a protuberant face. Neanderthals used tools similar to those of early *H. sapiens*. While their capacities and capabilities can only be indirectly inferred, there is some anatomical evidence, such as the size of the hypoglossal foramen and the shape of the hyoid bone, which suggests some ability for vocalization. There is also some scanty and controversial evidence for carving and artistic representation which may have been copied from co-existent *H. sapiens*. There is evidence that at least 70 000 years ago Neanderthals buried their dead and that this was associated with defleshment, which might represent some form of ritual.

DNA evidence suggests that the lineage giving rise to *H. sapiens* and to Neanderthals diverged about 450 000 years ago from a later lineage of the *H. erectus* line, now often called *H. heidelbergensis* or archaic *H. sapiens*. The evolution of *H. sapiens* involved a decrease in robustness of the face and skeleton and a progressive change in functional capacities associated with locomotion, behaviour, social organization, and culture. It is now clear from molecular studies that this change occurred only in Africa, with other populations of *H. erectus* and successor species such as *H. neanderthalensis* eventually becoming extinct. Anatomically modern humans appeared in eastern Africa approximately 160 000–200 000 years ago and remained localized to that continent until about 100 000 years ago. The use of mitochondrial DNA and Y-chromosomal mapping has allowed the reconstruction of subsequent migrations of humans from Africa to

be studied in considerable detail (see below). That dispersion plays a major role in understanding the origins of human diversity.

Climate change leading to ecological change and progressive deforestation in eastern Africa clearly played a major role in our development from an arboreal ancestor into a bipedal terrestrial ape. The evidence suggests that over the last 5 million years there have been a number of cycles of warming and cooling. Of particular relevance are major cooling events about 5 MYA, and again between 3.5 and 2.5 MYA, which led to a major build-up of polar ice. At about this time the Panamanian isthmus rose and joined the Americas, altering patterns of circulation in the oceans. Many other major climate events leading to changing ocean levels and environments occurred in the subsequent 2.5 million years and played a role in allowing humans to migrate around the globe. The range of the Neanderthal was restricted by the glaciations that occupied northern and middle Europe from approximately

---

Box 6.1   Is there a Neanderthal in all of us?

The Human Genome Project passed a significant milestone when the sequence of the last chromosome was published in May 2006. Several groups are now attempting to sequence components of the Neanderthal genome, and a complete sequence is expected soon. The sequence of Neanderthal mitochondrial DNA has already been published, using DNA extracted from a 38 000-year-old Neanderthal femur discovered in Croatia. Human and Neanderthal mitochondrial DNAs differ at more than 200 positions out of the 16 565 bases examined, while modern humans differ at only about 100 positions when compared with each other; these numbers suggest that humans and Neanderthals diverged more than 600 000 years ago. Early results for the Neanderthal nuclear genome suggest 99.5% genetic identity with modern humans and divergence dates ranging from 500 000 to 800 000 years ago.

But what of the popular hypothesis that Neanderthals and modern humans interbred freely?

A particular problem in analysing the Neanderthal genome is contamination with modern human DNA, which would tend to cause underestimation of the difference between the genomes. Studies of Neanderthal DNA are being very careful to avoid human DNA contamination during sample preparation and analysis, and so far no evidence of admixture with human genetic material has been found, suggesting that interbreeding did not occur. But there is an intriguing hint of such an event from an unrelated study. The most common form of the microcephalin gene in modern humans (microcephalin regulates brain size, and has been under strong selection in the human lineage; see Box 6.4, below) appears to result from admixture (a process called **introgression**) with an archaic human lineage just 37 000 years ago. The timing of this introgression means that Neanderthals may be the candidate for that lineage.

Box 6.2 *Homo floresiensis?*

In September 2003, an archaeological expedition to the Liang Bua cave on the island of Flores, Indonesia, uncovered the skull and partial skeleton of an 18000-year-old hominin. Several other specimens have subsequently been found in the cave. Various primitive and derived features led the discoverers to denote the remains as a species distinct from *H. sapiens*. Named *Homo floresiensis* in recognition of its island of discovery, the skeleton was determined to be that of an adult female who was just 1 m in stature. This, the researchers postulated, was a consequence of dwarfing of an ancestral *H. erectus* population on Flores. Inevitably, the popular press dubbed these hominins 'hobbits'. Besides its extremely small physical size, what stood out about the skeleton was its very small brain volume (≈ 380 cm^3 compared to ≈ 980 cm^3

for late *H. erectus* and ≈ 1350 cm^3 for modern humans). Given the presence of sophisticated stone tools at the site, other researchers have argued that the specimen could well be a small-bodied and microcephalic modern human. Yet others have argued that the remains are of *H. sapiens* affected by endemic cretinism because of low iodine levels. Supporters of *H. floresiensis* cite unusual anatomical features of the skeletons, traditional stories of small-bodied people in the area, and evidence for persistence of *H. erectus* in island South-east Asia until less than 30000 years ago. Unfortunately, it is unlikely that DNA can be recovered from the putative *H. floresiensis* remains. Controversy still rages regarding the true nature of *H. floresiensis*, although the majority of evidence supports a distinct *Homo* species.

100000 to 10000 years ago. The late stage of the last glacial period 12000 years ago may have allowed grasses to grow in the Middle East, promoting the development of agriculture. The changing nature of food supply meant a shift from an exclusively herbaceous diet to a mixed diet, first by scavenging and then by hunting. Clearly there was selective advantage in the development and use of technology: group living, communication, and cultural capacities both reinforced and were reinforced by these factors.

6.3.2 Bipedalism

By about 4 MYA, *Australopithecus* was a generally bipedal hominoid and facultative bipedalism may have been present in even earlier species. Fossil hallmarks of bipedalism include the positioning of the foramen magnum, which becomes more central as the posture becomes more upright and the skull must be supported by the spinal column. There are also changes in the shape of the pelvis, hip socket, and femora. There have been many hypotheses put forward, and entire books written, regarding the adaptive origins of bipedalism, some compromised by an

anthropocentric and even teleological tendency to think of humans as special.

Human bipedalism has features which are distinct from the occasional bipedalism of other apes. The knee is very different, allowing the leg to straighten and the knee to lock, minimizing energy expenditure in supporting the body when standing upright. Humans have a pelvic and muscular structure which allows the centre of gravity to shift only slightly on each step, whereas species such as the chimpanzee waddle because an enormous shift in the centre of gravity occurs on each step. Being able to walk this way has meant the evolution of a differently shaped pelvis and an angled femur and a change in the limb-moving muscles such as the gluteal abductors. Humans can run, a development which first became anatomically possible in early *Homo* species. We are thought to be unique in being able to undertake endurance running, as well as sprinting, which perhaps allowed us to hunt down prey.

It is generally accepted that the origins of bipedalism were associated with the shift from an arboreal to a more open environment in East Africa about 4 MYA. Perhaps the most favoured hypothesis is that this environmental shift was associated with food resources becoming more dispersed across these open habitats. In such habitats, bipedal movement is energetically more effective than quadripedal movement, particularly at walking speeds. The palaeoanthropologist Robert Foley has calculated that, provided the early hominid spent the majority of its time in terrestrial (as opposed to arboreal) foraging, then bipedalism would be adaptive in such environments. Thus the evolution of bipedalism can be seen to have been progressively adaptive as the hominin line evolved, driven by habitat change.

Other arguments that have been put forward for the origin of bipedalism include better thermoregulatory efficiency – being upright exposes less of the body to the sun. This would significantly reduce the demand for fluids. The loss of body hair has also been suggested as a component of this thermoregulatory adaptation as it would allow more effective sweat evaporation. Both these adaptations would allow foraging to extend through the heat of the day.

Others have suggested that being upright allows greater capacity for predator avoidance by allowing the individual to see further, just as the meerkat stands upright when on guard. It has also been suggested that it allows the hominid to carry things better, including foods, tools, and children during their long infantile period. While these arguments have much popular appeal, they are more likely to be secondary exaptations (see Chapter 2) which arose from and amplified the initial adaptation of standing upright and adopting a bipedal gait.

However, bipedalism has costs. The most obvious is back pain, which is one of the most common reasons for consulting a doctor. The shift from a quadripedal to an upright posture came late in the evolutionary history of primates and the accommodation reached in terms of a lumbar lordosis creates pressure on the intervertebral discs and the sacroiliac joints. Prolapse of a disc, with injury to the lumbar nerves innervating the lower limbs, leads to pain, paraesthesia, and sometimes motor dysfunction. Such problems are aggravated by being overweight, putting even greater pressure on the intervertebral discs, and by osteoarthritis and osteoporosis, problems of advanced age characteristic of the post-industrial modern human. The upright posture makes injurious falls more likely as people age, because their gait and balance become more unsteady and they have failing vision. As

they develop osteopenia the risk of femoral neck fractures becomes very high; the mortality associated with femoral neck fracture is a major concern in the older population. The shape of the pelvis is changed by an upright posture, necessitating a flattening of the pelvis and a change in the shape of the pelvic canal. As we will discuss in Chapter 7, many of the potential complications of human childbirth are consequential to this change.

6.3.3 Body size

The Australopithecines were small, ranging in weight from 18 to 45 kg, whereas *Homo* species were larger: their size reached a peak with early *H. sapiens*. It is not clear why body size increased over the course of hominin evolution. Clearly a number of countervailing evolutionary pressures were at work. Perhaps living in a more open environment exposed early hominins to a greater predation risk and so there was selection for larger individuals. There are costs to this increase in body size: the resulting increase in metabolic rate (see Chapter 5) required hominids with their mixed diets to expand their home range for foraging. The alternative approach is to become adapted to eating large quantities of low caloric foods: this is the strategy of the gorilla which has a small foraging range but requires a large intestinal system to digest the large amounts of plant material it ingests. The increase in body size would cause greater problems in thermoregulation which may have been ameliorated by upright posture and loss of body hair. The time to reach adult maturity took longer and living in social groups thus became a key feature for care and protection. The presence of larger social groups allowed a greater feeding range to be occupied. Energy requirements would have been further exacerbated by the high energetic demands of a relatively large brain.

6.3.4 Face, jaw, and dentition

There were major changes in the face, jaw, and dentition as the hominoid line evolved. In general, hominins evolved a flatter face with the jaw less protuberant and the teeth tucked under the face relative to modern apes. Thus there is a progressive change in mandibular shape to the modern L shape. Humans have much less developed masseter muscles compared to their early forebears and this is associated with other skeletal changes such as a smaller zygomatic arch. These changes suggest that a less powerful chewing action was needed by later-evolving hominin species and this became even more so once fire became used to cook meat. The first evidence for controlled use of fire (hearths, earth ovens, and charred animal bones) dates to about 500 000 years ago.

The change in jaw shape allowed for a more grinding type of mastication and this was associated with a change in dentition. The incisors became less prominent compared with those of other primates and the molars became larger. These changes reflect a difference in diet from the purely fruit-based diet of apes to a more omnivorous diet. There is evidence that when in recent centuries human infants began to be fed on particularly soft foods, the need for grinding movements become less, and the risk of dental malocclusion increased. The flattening of the face and the change in posture also changed the positioning of the eustachian tubes. This contributes to the risks of otitis media. The changes in the position of the larynx associated with vocalization are associated with increased risk of obstructive apnoea, especially during sleep.

6.3.5 Gastrointestinal tract

The earliest primates were insectivores, and as they became larger they became herbivores. There are some modern primates such as the langur which have large stomachs, analogous to the ruminant stomach, to allow bacterial digestion of cellulose in the upper gut. But most herbivores rely on slow intestinal transit and ileo-caecal digestion. A large caecum is typical of such an intestinal system that needs to digest high-fibre food. As the diet shifts from a frugivorous nature to a more omnivorous diet, a very long gastrointestinal tract and a large caecum become energetically inefficient.

The earliest hominins were exclusive herbivores but relied primarily on fruits and tubers rather than on the high-cellulose diets typical of leaf- and grass-eaters. The later Australopithecines probably also scavenged for meat, and meat became a larger component of the *Homo* diet, particularly once fire was adopted for cooking. As noted above, these changes are reflected in the jaw and dentition as well as in the gastrointestinal tract. The appendix is an atavistic reminder of our evolutionary

origin as a frugivore. Indeed, Darwin recognized it to be a rudimentary or vestigial organ, there being no evidence that the appendix has unique functions, even though it does contain some lymphoid tissue. Appendicitis is the outcome of this vestigial organ becoming infected: it is prone to inflammation and rupture. Appendicitis can be fatal and its peak incidence occurs in adolescence and early adulthood, so it is interesting to speculate why there has not been more active selection against it. The evidence is that appendicitis was rare until recently: its prevalence appears to have risen in the nineteenth and early twentieth centuries in developed countries, where its incidence is now declining again; the incidence is much lower in traditional and less developed societies. Thus there would be little selection pressure operating on this vestigial organ. While the reasons for the association between modern development and appendicitis are unclear, they are likely to be related to changes in intestinal flora or the presence (or lack) of intestinal parasites.

6.3.6 The hairless ape

All other primates, including the other apes, are fully covered with hair except for the palms of their hands and feet. It is not known when hominins lost this characteristic. The most generally held explanation is that the hair loss aided thermoregulation, even though all other primates living in tropical climates are fully haired. An alternative thesis would hold that hairlessness does not have an adaptive origin through natural selection but may have evolved by sexual selection. When a feature appears rapidly and uniquely in one species within a clade, sexual selection needs to be considered as a possible explanation. The retention of pubic hair in both sexes and of facial hair in males might support this argument. Pubic hair only appears at puberty and in both sexes the full pattern of sexual hair would be a sign of sexual maturity. Similarly, facial hair may serve this purpose in the male and breast development and the appearance of menses could do so in the female.

6.3.7 The hominin brain

Figure 6.2 shows the change in brain volume calculated from fossil skull dimensions across the hominin lineage. Brain size, in both absolute terms and relative to body

---

Box 6.3   The missing vitamin

The atmosphere contains 21% oxygen, and humans get their energy by using this oxygen to oxidize nutrients within their cells. But at the beginning of life 3.6 billion years ago, the atmosphere contained no oxygen. The oxygen now essential to animal life comes from photosynthesis by plants, and thus significant amounts of oxygen first appeared in the atmosphere with the evolution of photosynthesis about 2 billion years ago.

Our oxygen-based metabolism is not an unmitigated blessing. Oxygen is fiercely reactive and oxygen-derived by-products of cell metabolism, called reactive oxygen species (ROS), are toxic to tissues. The amounts of ROS produced are not negligible and organisms have developed defence mechanisms against ROS. These include enzymes that detoxify ROS as well as antioxidants that react with and scavenge ROS. Because the chemical processes of photosynthesis are a particularly rich source of ROS, plants have developed a wide array of antioxidants to protect themselves from the deleterious effects of these ROS: compounds such as carotenoids, flavenoids, tocopherols (vitamin E), and ascorbic acid (vitamin C) are all found in abundance in plants.

Since plants are rich in antioxidants, animals have lost the ability to synthesize many of them and rely on dietary sources for their supply of these compounds. For most vertebrates the exception is vitamin C, which they can synthesize. Vitamin C is a powerful antioxidant and has another essential function as a cofactor in the synthesis of collagen, a major structural component of connective tissue. Yet humans, along with other primates and, peculiarly, guinea pigs among a very few other mammals, cannot synthesize vitamin C and must obtain it from their diet. The reason is a frameshift mutation in the gene for the last enzyme of the vitamin C biosynthetic pathway, which renders the enzyme non-functional. As a result, humans require at least 10 mg of vitamin C daily in their diet, and failure to obtain this amount is first apparent clinically as an inability to repair connective tissue, causing the symptoms of scurvy.

Why is it that primates have lost the ability to synthesize this essential cofactor? Probably for the same reasons that mammals have lost the ability to synthesize other plant-based antioxidants: because vitamin C is abundant and available for free in the fruit-rich diets of many primates, including those from which the great ape and human lineage eventually evolved. Another possibility is that, as for other apparently deleterious mutations such as those responsible for sickle cell anaemia, there might be some benefit conferred by an inability to synthesis vitamin C. Although numerous 'benefit' theories have been proposed, the most likely explanation is that there was little selection to maintain endogenous synthesis in a dietary niche in which vitamin C is abundant.

---

size, did not change dramatically in the earliest members of the lineage. Australopithecines had absolute and relative brain sizes not greatly different from those of the modern apes. Brain size expansion started with the appearance of *Homo* species and showed an exponential increase from *habilis*, through *erectus* to *neanderthalensis*, and then a slight decrease to *sapiens*. During this period, average brain volume increased from about 400 to 1250 cm³. This can be expressed as the encephaliza-tion quotient (EQ) which is an allometric calculation of the relationship between brain mass and body mass (in mammals the most widely used formula is $EQ = $ brain weight $/ 0.12$(body weight)$^{2/3}$).

The common chimpanzee has an EQ of 2.0, Australopithecines had an EQ of about 2.5, *H. erectus* an EQ of about 3.3, and modern *H. sapiens* has an EQ of 5.8. As hominoid body size has generally increased through this lineage, the enhanced encephalization suggests

---

Box 6.5 A lousy way of determining when humans started to wear clothing

Two factors are likely to have initiated the use of clothing by hominids: loss of insulating body hair and migration resulting in exposure to cooler climates. The archaeological evidence for the origin of clothing is scant, since furs and fibres do not preserve well. The oldest tools associated with the manufacture of clothing, bone needles, date from about 40 000 years ago, although there are much older examples of scrapers that might have been used to clean an animal pelt.

An innovative approach to finding an answer came from studies on the molecular genetics of the human louse (*Pediculus humanus*). There are two subspecies of this parasite: the head louse feeds exclusively on the scalp and attaches its eggs to hairs, while the body louse feeds on the body and attaches its eggs to clothing. It's a reasonable assumption that the two subspecies began to diverge at the time humans began to wear clothing. Molecular clock analysis of DNA sequences from head and body lice suggests a divergence date of around 100 000 years ago, which the authors of the study described as 'surprisingly recent'.

---

there was a further expansion in the range of stone tools made in Europe, coincident with the other evidence of cultural development including representative art, carvings, and decorative items such as beads. This is the period when modern humans displaced the Neanderthal, and is termed the **Upper Palaeolithic revolution**.

6.3.9 Language

One of the most contentious debates in human evolutionary biology is over the timing of the evolution of the capacity for language. The informed views range in dating this from early *Homo* some 400 000 years ago to its appearing as recently as 50 000 years ago. The difficulty is the limited anatomical substrates which can be used to infer language, since the soft tissues of the larynx are not preserved as fossils. The scanty anatomical evidence suggests that some form of vocalization was possible in early *Homo*. The other major form of evidence has been inference from the study of material (such as tools and artefacts) and social structure and behaviour. It has been suggested, for example, that relatively consistent patterns of tool-making, some of which involved quite complex but arbitrary patterns of design, imply the use of language for their transmission. A stronger argument can be derived from studies of the development of art, rituals, and social rules. The first evidence of symbolic art may date to some rudimentary markings in the Blombos cave

in South Africa estimated to be about 70 000 years old. But unequivocal representative art in the form of cave paintings or carved figures dates to only about 35 000 years ago in Europe and perhaps as early as 50 000 years ago in Australia. Some of this art, particularly in Australia, clearly involves use of abstraction and suggests the capacity for thought, which is intimately related to language capacity.

Language is generally considered to have evolved as a way of assisting communication within the social group. Cooperative ventures such as hunting would be aided by such communication, although many other species such as wolves can cooperate in hunting without requiring advanced language. Indeed, there has been a shift in emphasis towards viewing the evolution of language in a different context: namely to aid the capacity to be conscious and to analyse the perceived world. It is widely believed that it is not possible to build a construct of the world beyond the immediate present without language in some form. Dunbar has gone further in arguing that language was key to the maintenance of larger stable social groups of the order of 150 individuals which characterized our ancestral social organization, and to some extent still do (Table 6.1). Whereas grooming is used to achieve social cohesion in other primate organizational groups, language would have been a more effective and efficient means of doing so as social groups became larger and the capacity for grooming across the full community became

Table 6.1 Examples of human social groupings. All cluster around the 'Dunbar number' of 150 predicted from human brain size.

Grouping	Size
Neolithic villages (Middle East, 7500–6500 years before present)	150–200
Roman army maniple 'double century' (2000 years before present)	120–130
Average English village size (Domesday book, 1086)	150
Average English village size (eighteenth century)	160
Tribal societies (mean and range of nine communities)	148 (90–222)
Hunter-gatherer societies (mean of 213 clans)	165
Hutterite farming communities in Canada (mean of 51)	107
Amish parishes in Nebraska (mean of 8)	113
Church congregations (recommended ideal size, 1974)	200
East Tennessee rural mountain community	197
Social network size (mean of 2)	134
Clothing factory unit size	150
Military company (mean and range for 10 armies in World War 2)	180 (124–223)
Christmas card distribution lists (mean of 43)	154

Modified from Dunbar, R.I.M. (2008) *British Academy Reviews* **11**, 15–17, with permission.

limited by time. There is thus a loose interaction between social group structure, brain size, and language, and while it is not possible to be definitive, the weight of evidence suggests that language evolved relatively recently, perhaps 70 000 years ago. In turn this supported and reinforced our social organization and allowed the development of a more complex mental world which could support the development of art, music, belief, and political systems.

Equally contentious, in the area of evolutionary psychology is the substrate of language evolution. There are basically two schools of thought: one holds that language is an incidental outcome of developing a large brain and is largely derived from cultural evolution; the other maintains that language evolved specifically through selection.

Some notable theorists, including Stephen Jay Gould, have adhered to the first school and argued that the substrates for language did not evolve through natural selection. Gould considered that language evolved because of cultural possibilities arising from possessing something biologically like a general-purpose computer. This view is not generally accepted, but seems to have been a response to both the enthusiasm for finding an adaptationist explanation for every phenomenon and because of the position which Gould took up in the sociobiology debate (see Chapter 10), namely to argue against evolutionary explanations for much of human behaviour.

The leading theorist for the other camp – a selective origin of language – is Steven Pinker. There is little doubt that hominins evolved with specific features enabling them to speak and use language (e.g. the shape of the larynx, Broca's and Wernicke's areas in the neocortex). There is evidence for these features even in early species of *Homo*. Thus the 'design' argument would maintain that active selection for language occurred. Pinker would argue that language is the key reason why hominins developed a large brain, and this implies that proto-language developed in early *Homo* species. It is easy to envisage adaptive advantage with even the minimal capacity for vocalization and then symbolic language. Further there are genetic abnormalities that affect speech and grammar (see Box 6.6) and this is an argument for genetic determinants and thus selection on the capacity to use language. Young children acquire language very easily, suggesting an innate ability from a (genetic and selected) substrate which underpins the capacity to develop use of the rules of language – in this regard it is important to recognize that infants learn fluent, grammatically correct language by passive exposure rather than by being formally taught grammatical rules and syntax. This in turn leads to another debate (beyond the scope of this book) as to whether there is a universal grammar with a genetic substrate underpinning it: it is a debate which keeps linguistic research lively.

Box 6.6 Can the genetic basis for speech and grammar tell us about when language evolved?

Dyslexia is a neurobehavioural disorder where an individual of normal intelligence experiences difficulty with reading, writing, and spelling. Mutations in 'reading disorder' genes, such as *DCDC2* on chromosome 6 and *ROBO1* on chromosome 3, together account for more than one in five cases of dyslexia.

Studies of a large family with severe impairment of language ability identified a causative point mutation in another gene, *FOXP2*. This codes for a transcription factor able to regulate the expression of multiple target genes. Unfortunately, this resulted in the popular press proclaiming *FOXP2* as a 'language gene'. Language is complex and clearly not reliant on any single gene. However, from an evolutionary perspective what is important is that the underlying genetic basis for these disorders supports the proposal that development of language was selected for during human evolution.

Human FOXP2 is a transcription factor that consists of 715 amino acids; it differs from that of mice by three amino acids and from that of chimpanzees, gorillas, and rhesus macaques by two. The high rate of divergence after the human/chimpanzee divergence is suggestive of a role of FOXP2 in human language evolution. Neanderthal FOXP2 also possesses the same two mutations as modern humans; it remains uncertain whether Neanderthals had the capacity for language.

6.3.10 Culture and society

H. sapiens is a social animal. We live in groups and there is considerable evidence that our ancestor hominids also did so. Figure 6.4 illustrates the concept that there is a relationship between brain size and group size within primates. It has been deduced from this relationship that the pre-agricultural human group comprised between 50 and 150 individuals. We are adapted to living in groups which requires cooperation and adherence to rules and customs; in turn this is dependent on reciprocal altruism and overt ways of dealing with 'freeloaders', individuals who take from but do not contribute to the group. Much of human behaviour can be understood in terms of the requirements for successfully living in such a social structure.

'Culture' is an amalgam of knowledge, behaviour, and tradition within a particular community or population. It can be manifest in technology and tools, in art and music, in belief, myth, stories, and tradition, in behaviour, and in social structure and organization. There is an intimate relationship between our biological and cultural evolution. There are, however, two cultural factors which have played a major role in defining modern human life and its impact on our health: the development of agriculture and the development of towns. The earliest modern *H. sapiens* lived as mobile small bands of foragers. They moved to find new food supplies if there were ecological changes that affected their environment. As populations grew they would have dispersed across wider and wider geographical areas and the environments to which they had to adapt became more diverse. But *H. sapiens* achieved a capacity to control its environment through fire, tools, clothing, and buildings. It is this innovative capacity which made, and still makes, humans such an effective generalist species.

Agriculture developed independently in several geographical areas. Its earliest appearance was in the Levant of the Middle East about 11 000 years ago, and independent developments appeared about 5000 years ago in sub-Saharan Africa, in parts of North and South America, and more recently in New Guinea. The adoption of agriculture was a gradual process, and whether it preceded or followed the development of the first villages is unclear. There is, for example, evidence of a village in northern Syria which was settled some 11 500 years ago, prior to

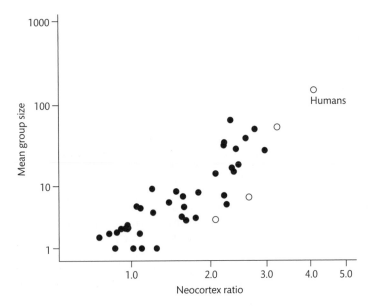

Figure 6.4 Mean social group size for different species of primate plotted against relative neocortex volume (neocortex volume divided by the volume of the rest of the brain). Ape species are shown as open symbols; the human point is predicted from the ape regression equation (from Dunbar, R.I.M. (2008) *British Academy Review* **11**, 15–17, with permission).

evidence of agriculture; this may have been a traditional forager clan which, while living in one place, was able to forage locally for abundant wild cereals and hunt game. There were similar historical forager societies in British Columbia which lived as sedentary groups in villages because food was plentiful locally.

Climate change may have played a role in the development of agriculture. The cooler conditions in Mesopotamia 12000 years ago would have promoted wild cereal growth and attracted game and this would have allowed the adoption of a sedentary lifestyle. The development of an agricultural lifestyle implies a degree of social complexity to allow the organization of both pastoralism and crop care. So there is a direct link between the evolution of agriculture and the shift to living in villages.

These changes had profound implications for the health of our species. First there was a progressive change in diet: as plants were artificially selected to allow for planting and cultivation, the balance of foods changed. Herding, at least in some societies, allowed the collection of milk as a food source as well as access to meat on a more consistent basis. The domestication of animals brought humans into much closer contact with them and so an increased risk of infectious disease. Many viral, bacterial, and parasitic diseases such as influenza and

tuberculosis have their origin in domestic animal hosts (see Chapter 9). Further, as populations became sedentary and lost the capacity to forage, they became more at mercy of drought, floods, and crop failure. Malnutrition and disease thus paradoxically become a greater risk with the development of agriculture. Larger cities created problems of hygiene which reached catastrophic proportions in Europe by the nineteenth century.

Second, settlement brought a drastic change in the way we live. Groups of people now would live in a common place and, as these groups got larger, skills started to be separated in society and a group structure with traditions, rules, and beliefs was required. Political structures had to be developed. The tendency to urbanization, complex social structures, and differentiation of social roles has continued unabated since that time. As we shall discuss in Chapter 10, this in turn creates pressures on our capacity to cope and may play a major role in the origin of mental disorders as well as impacting on our physical health.

As society became more complex and formalized, political and formal religious systems evolved. Religion probably first evolved informally as a way for our prescient species to explain natural phenomena and perhaps to propitiate against possible future disasters. As belief became a central component of social organization for a group, enshrined in ritual and in special knowledge held

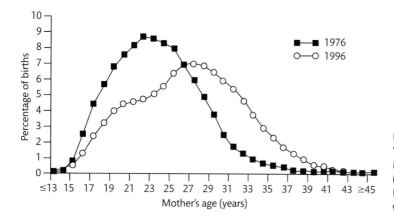

Figure 6.5 Rapidity of cultural evolution. The peak age of first birth in Canada increased by 5 years from 1976 to 1996 (modified from Health Canada, Health Policy Research Bulletin, Issue 10, May 2005, with permission).

by shamans, the capacity for religion to become a social controlling force became apparent. Thus religion and political power became linked. The beginnings of medicine are linked very much to the evolution of religious belief: the power of healing being linked to shamanism, special knowledge, and invocation of the supernatural. Healing gods became a focus for, and their priests the providers of, primitive medicines.

6.3.11 Cultural evolution

With the development of the capacity to communicate, observe, and learn comes the potential for a different mode of inter-individual and inter-generational transmission of information: **cultural inheritance**. This is not restricted to humans, since other species show the capacity to adopt behaviours. For example, the ability of blue tits to open the foil tops of traditional British milk bottles spread rapidly when these tops were introduced. It is unlikely that each bird initiated the skill *de novo*; rather, many would have gained the skill from observation of others.

There has been considerable study of cultural transmission in non-human primates. One classic example is that of potato washing in macaques on a Japanese island. Scientists were in the habit of placing potatoes on a sandy beach to attract the animals out of the forest. Once one female macaque had learned to remove sand from her potatoes by washing them in the sea, other monkeys and eventually all the monkeys in the troop adopted the same behaviour. Chimpanzees in different parts of Africa use sticks to extract termites, but they do so in quite different ways reflecting different cultural traditions within the different troops.

In contradistinction to genetic inheritance, cultural inheritance need not involve vertical transmission between generations. Horizontal transmission is the norm; for example, when young people adopt a particular form of dress we can see that it is rapidly transmitted through the peer group. But culture itself undergoes evolution. Every aspect of human culture from belief, to art, language, music, and technology shows a process of change which is termed **cultural evolution**. There is variation in a culturally determined characteristic and there will be selection by the society as to which variants are preferred and thus which become successfully spread. However, the fidelity of replication need not be sustained, unlike most genetic replication for which there are repair mechanisms which generally maintain fidelity. Thus change can be rapid: witness how quickly the change in the age when women choose to have their first child became distributed across Western society (Figure 6.5).

The term 'cultural evolution' implies some similarities with biological evolution. Indeed, at a superficial level there are similarities, and this led to development of the concept of **memes**, a term first introduced by Richard Dawkins. As initially proposed, memes were true units of cultural inheritance, capable of self replication, with variation due to errors in duplication, and which due to the nature of a society would have differential 'reproductive' success (in other words a kind of fitness for memes, how well they persisted and spread within a population). But this concept is now seen by most evolutionary psychologists as nothing more than a useful metaphor.

The very nature of culture means that its specific manifestations are not genetically determined, although the capacity to exhibit culture must have a genetic basis. For example, as is discussed in Chapter 7, the 'acting out' behaviour of young males, whether on the sports field or in driving fast cars, has its origin in the evolved determinants of male behaviour related to displaying evidence of relative fitness, the result of sexual selection. Culture itself unconsciously affects fitness: it generates behaviours which promote potential reproductive success for the individual through creating rules for membership of a group and promoting reciprocal altruistic behaviour (examples being religion and food sharing) or which allow the potential reproductive value of the individual to be demonstrated (for example, art and fashion).

Cultural evolution can influence biological evolution and vice versa: this phenomenon is known as **gene/culture co-evolution**. Consider the example with which we introduced this book, lactose intolerance. Only those with the genetic variant allowing for lactase persistence could nutritionally thrive on a diet including cow's milk.

When certain populations domesticated cattle those individuals thrived and the population underwent selection for the persistence of the allele. In turn, as the population became more able to utilize dairy products, farming of cattle would be promoted. The presence of the heterozygote state for sickle cell anaemia confers protection against malaria. Changes in farming practice in West Africa led to more stagnant pools of water, and thus a higher incidence of malaria, and this may have favoured in turn an increase in gene frequency of an allele conferring relative protection against malaria. So we can see how interactions between inherited culture and genetic variation can shape human evolution.

Humans create their own environments. Their capacities to make clothing, to use fire and to build shelter are examples of ways in which we use our technological capacity to allow us to survive and flourish in a variety of environments. Many other species create a built environment in which they breed and generally live: the termite's nest is brilliantly designed by the colony to maintain a constant internal temperature and the beaver's nest provides both protection and a constant environment in which to breed. In most species such niche construction

---

Box 6.7 Studying cultural evolution

Culture is predicted to undergo evolution in much the same way as genetic evolution, where cultural features that are tested against the environment evolve at a different rate to those not tested against the environment. However, using a scientific framework to support this has been difficult since humans tend to be unpredictable in their beliefs and behaviours. A recent study on Polynesian canoe designs provides empirical evidence for this argument. The researchers found that a large data set characterizing detailed features of canoes was available, and set about examining a total of 134 functional and symbolic features. A functional trait would, for example, be whether canoes were made up from a single trunk or several, or whether they were sewn together from coconut fibres. These

features would have been important in the seaworthiness of the canoes and thus the survival of their builders. Symbolic traits examined included paintings and shell decorations, which have no impact on the canoe's sturdiness. Statistical analysis showed that functional traits evolved more slowly than symbolic traits, indicating that features that improved survival, migration, and reproduction tended to be preserved. This is a manifestation of the adage that 'if it ain't broke, don't fix it'. Thus in a way, natural selection was acting to prevent persistence of inferior designs. More importantly, it demonstrated that evolution of culture can be measured, and that this process can indeed be considered akin to the way natural selection operates in genetic evolution.

is stereotypic and is likely to be genetically determined, possibly having arisen through genetic assimilation (see Chapter 4). Humans could be considered as niche constructors but they do not produce a stereotypic niche; rather, they use their technological and innovative capacity to find ways to modify their environments, expanding the environmental range in which they can live.

6.4 Human adaptation to local selection pressures

6.4.1 Hominin origins and migrations: out of Africa again

Archaeological, molecular genetic, and linguistic data are now sufficient to document with reasonable certainty the origin and dispersal of modern humans. It is clear that there have been two major dispersals of *Homo* species from Africa within the last million years. As described in section 6.3.1, *H. erectus* spread out of Africa into Asia about 1 MYA and their descendants *H. neanderthalensis* populated Europe from about 400 000 years ago up to about 30 000 years ago. *H. sapiens* evolved from *H. erectus* in East Africa between 200 000 and 160 000 years ago, but remained largely restricted to that continent for many millennia until about 60 000–70 000 years ago, when a relatively small group of those people departed from eastern Africa across the mouth of the Red Sea. They became the founder population for all modern humans living outside Africa.

Genetic evidence (see Box 6.8, below) points to a sub-Saharan African origin of anatomically modern humans, and indeed the genetic lineages found in the Khoisan people of South-western Africa (also known as the ¡Kung san: we will meet them again in Chapter 8 as prototypical hunter-gatherers) provide evidence that they are among the oldest human populations. Human mitochondrial DNA lineages coalesce about 140 000 years ago, or in other words they can be traced to a single woman who lived at that time, a finding that prompted much media comment about 'mitochondrial Eve'. Naturally, this does not mean she was the only woman living at the time. Women who have only male offspring do not pass on their mitochondrial DNA and there will have been many other women living at the time of 'Eve' although their genetic legacy, at least in the form of mitochondrial

DNA, has been lost. Studies of Y-chromosome variation point to a somewhat later coalescence: the apparent discrepancy may be the result of a smaller effective population size (see Chapter 3) in males possibly arising from the socio-cultural phenomenon where, in many traditional societies, a few dominant men father most of the children.

During the period of about 100 000 years between the emergence of modern humans and the beginning of their worldwide expansion, the *H. sapiens* population in Africa appears to have lived in small and geographically isolated groups that had only begun to mix towards the end of that time. The event that precipitated the out-of-Africa migration will probably always remain unknown, but displacement by some form of intergroup rivalry is a possibility. Certainly the departing group was relatively few in number, because they carried only a small proportion of African genetic diversity. Remarkably, of the 40–50 human matrilineal lineages (as assessed by analysis of mitochondrial DNA) that existed in Africa at the time of the out-of-Africa event, only two (for the record, they are known as L3M and L3N) actually contribute to worldwide non-African diversity. Similarly, all non-African Y chromosomes carry the mutation M168. This founder effect means that modern African populations carry the highest amount of human genetic diversity, and people in the regions last to be populated by modern humans, Western Europe, the Americas, and Oceania, carry the least.

Where did the African emigrants go? The world was colder 50 000 years ago, the icefields of the northern hemisphere had sequestered large amounts of water, sea levels were perhaps 100 m lower than today, and the coastlines of the continents stretched much farther out to sea than they do now, with some present-day islands forming single landmasses with the adjacent coasts. These conditions allowed human expansion around the tropical beaches of Southern and South-eastern Asia, and there is archaeological evidence for human presence in Australia by around 40 000 years ago. Another group appears to have headed northward through the Arabian peninsula to the Levant and Mesopotamia, thence spreading eastwards across the steppes of Central Asia to populate Siberia and, for those who travelled south of the Central Asian massif, India and eventually China. There is also evidence that some of the earlier coastal migrants moved

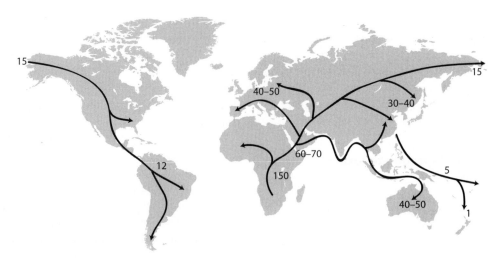

Figure 6.6 Routes of human migration. The routes and dates shown are composites of published mitochondrial DNA and Y-chromosome data. Numbers represent the time (thousands of years ago, KYA) when settlement was achieved.

northwards through South-east Asia, explaining the clear genetic differentiation between the northern and southern Han Chinese.

Thus by 35 000 years ago modern humans had populated essentially all of Africa and Asia (Figure 6.6). These modern humans may have encountered, and replaced, some remnant populations of the earlier migration out of Africa by *H. erectus* over a million years previously, as *H. erectus* fossils in Java may date from as little as 27 000 years ago. There is better support for encounters between two *Homo* species during the peopling of Europe by *H. sapiens* beginning 40 000 years ago, since there is strong archaeological evidence that some populations of *H. neanderthalensis* persisted in Western Europe up to 25 000–30 000 years ago. That westward migration of modern humans into Europe appears to have come from two sources, primarily from central Asia via a route north of the Black Sea but also via a Mediterranean route from the Levant. Whatever the nature of the encounters between *H. sapiens* and *H. neanderthalensis*, they almost certainly made no biological contribution to modern humanity, judging from the recent publication of the complete mitochondrial DNA sequence from *H. neanderthalensis*, revealing distinct differences between the species and a most recent common ancestor dating from much earlier, at least 500 000 years ago (but see Box 6.1).

The Americas were populated relatively recently by humans, probably no earlier than 15 000 years ago. The most commonly accepted model is that of one or more migrations by relatively small groups of Siberian hunters over the landmass called Beringia, joining present-day Siberia and Alaska, which existed from about 20 000 to 8000 years ago because of the fall in sea level during the last glacial period. The North American glaciers began to melt about 15 000 years ago, opening the way for a southward migration that reached the tip of South America 1000 years later. The original founding population was very small. The low genetic diversity of native Americans has caused some investigators to propose an effective population size for the migrating group of no more than 70 individuals (but remember that, for the reasons explained in Chapter 3, effective population size always underestimates true population size). An example of this low diversity is the low frequency of blood type A, and the virtual absence of blood type B, in native American populations.

The requirement for advanced technologies to enable humans to cross oceans meant that the last part of the world to be populated by *H. sapiens* was Oceania. Current theories of the peopling of Oceania suggest a southward and eastward migration of the Taiwanese Austronesian culture, beginning around 5500 years ago and reaching the last significant landmass, New Zealand, around 900 years ago.

suggest that pair bonding rather than extreme polygyny was more often the norm for humans. But the ethnographic data are mixed. Many cultures permit polygamy, serial monogamy is a common human behaviour, and mating outside the pair bond is not infrequent. Pair bonding has obvious advantages in ensuring resources for the offspring, and polygamy is less common where the male does not have adequate resources to support all his mates and offspring. Pair bonding may also be a form of mate guarding to ensure paternity: why would a male invest resources in an offspring not certain to be his? But once again perhaps cultural rather than evolutionary elements are the major drivers of monogamy to encourage successful living in family and social groups. Otherwise, the complex taboos which exist in many cultures may not have been required to reinforce it. This might suggest that the key evolutionary drivers of human mating behaviour related to our success in living in groups, and thus cultural factors, became critical in determining behavioural norms.

Individuals who are raised together up to the age of 5 years tend to have little sexual interest in each other. Similar effects can be seen in some other species. This phenomenon is known as the Westermarck effect. In most cases such closely reared infants are kin and so the risks of incest are reduced. The usual assumption has been that this process evolved to reduce the risks of inbreeding with consequent loss of genetic variation and accumulation of harmful mutations (inbreeding depression). In many species, such as the Malaysian tree shrew, matings will only occur between animals with distinct major histocompatibility (MHC) antigens. Many societies have taboos against incest which can be extremely complex. But exceptions are sometimes made, particularly for the rulers, and this may be related to safeguarding inheritance and as a way to prevent wealth accumulating outside the dominant family. Another argument is that these taboos encouraged marriage and alliances between clans which may have had advantages in ensuring access to key resources or reducing the risk of warfare.

Box 7.3   Homosexuality and celibacy

How can homosexuality be explained from an evolutionary perspective? This is a question which has assumed political overtones. Male–male or female–female genital contact or mounting behaviour is common in many species. It is observed even in parthenogenic species such as the New Mexican whiptail lizard which is an exclusively female species. But in sexual reproducing species within-gender sexual contact is essentially only seen in social species, and appears to be a way of reinforcing social bonds within a group: it has a significance not dissimilar to other social reinforcing behaviours such as grooming. The bonobo (sometimes known as the pygmy chimp) uses same-sex genital stimulation as well as heterosexual sexual behaviour as a way of maintaining social ties in a troop. Both same-sex and between-sex sexual behaviour is used by the bonobo to facilitate sharing of food, to promote reconciliation after a dispute, and to incorporate a newcomer into the troop. But in general across sexually reproducing species other than humans, same-sex sexual activity is never to the exclusion of heterosexual activity.

There has been considerable debate as to the presence of genetic factors associated with homosexuality in humans, and whether it has a developmental origin through either a biological or cultural process. For example, maternal exposure to stress in pregnancy or the nature of rearing have been variously suggested as possible factors. There is some evidence for differences in brain cell nuclei sizes in the hypothalamus between hetero- and homosexuals, but this need not have a causal or genetic basis and could be secondary to the development of the behaviour. Any genetic influence on homosexuality may have its origin in the selection of behaviours that promoted social behaviours and within-group bonding as observed in the bonobo.

However there can be no doubt that there is individual variation in sexual preference, whether of genetic, developmental, or social origin. Similarly there is little doubt that cultural factors such as social acceptance will determine the extent to which the activity is exhibited. Over history homosexuality has been viewed in various ways in different cultures but, in general, exclusive homosexuality has been relatively uncommon. The rapid change in social attitudes towards homosexuality in Western countries in recent years has allowed more people to exhibit their preference in sexual relationships, but this does not require a biological evolutionary explanation.

All the ancestors of all mammalian species alive today, including humans, have by definition engaged in heterosexual behaviour at least once. Thus there could not have been selection for exclusively homosexual behaviour. However, breeding activity and sexual preference must be distinguished; indeed, recent studies showed that the percentage of female homosexuals in the USA who were mothers was very similar to that of exclusively heterosexual women.

Celibacy may occur in males in many mammalian species where there is a dominant male mating system. But this is not voluntary or obligatory celibacy. The males who do not have a harem or achieve social dominance are striving to mate. They may do so by competition, dominance, or through surreptitious mating: the latter can be a highly effective strategy in some species such as rhesus macaques. But human societies, at least in historical times, contain individuals of either sex who elect a life of celibacy. In many cases this is linked to religious belief. In others it may also relate to maintaining economic wealth: the younger offspring of families in Medieval Europe entered the Church, not only for religious reasons but primarily to assist the economic development of their families. This could be interpreted as having some fitness value through kin selection.

7.7 Sexual differences in the human

Males and females are anatomically, physiologically, and behaviourally different. These sexually dimorphic characters are the result of both natural and sexual selection. One obvious difference between males and females is adult body size and muscle mass. The human male has a greater growth spurt at puberty and develops considerably more muscle mass. Humans demonstrate some sexual dimorphism in body size, although to a much lesser degree than the gorilla, suggesting that in our evolutionary history a partial-harem mating system was the norm. In some hunter-gatherer societies, mating rights are largely restricted to older men who take a number of younger female partners. Again this may be reflected in the differing ages of puberty.

Males tend to have delayed entry into puberty compared to females, there being no advantage to a male in having earlier puberty. Indeed, it may create a disadvantage in that the young male is immediately a potential reproductive threat to the older males. In many forager societies, females are viewed as reproductively competent and are married immediately after puberty. In contrast, male pubertal rites may involve long periods of exclusion or the development of rituals where the young males cannot mate for some years after sexual maturation. For example, the Masai tradition was for young adult males to become the soldiers for the tribe, and marriage was not possible until that period of effective sexual separation and exclusion had been completed. Even in Western society there are still echoes of these differences in our social structures.

In contrast to the marked physical evidence of sexual receptivity in the baboon which is signalled by a dramatic change in perineal coloration, human females have covert ovulation. It is speculated that covert ovulation evolved as a strategy to ensure that the male must attend to the female almost constantly to ensure other males do not get access. This would help reinforce the maternal-paternal-infant bond and thus ensure infant survival. Other explanations have also been put forward. If a male can detect when a female can ovulate then paternity may be more certain and this may lead to behaviours not in the mother's interests. In some species, such as the lion, a male may kill the offspring of a potential mate and another male. In humans, step-fathers are more likely to murder their step-children than their biological children. Thus greater certainty about paternity may lead to wasted resources, especially for the female.

Males and females have evolved a number of physical and behavioural characteristics which may reflect sexual selection. For example, human females have evolved large hips and pendular breasts, and males appear to have a sexual preference for women with an 'hour-glass' body shape. It is suggested that large breasts and pelvis may have been interpreted as surrogate markers of a capacity to give birth and to then nourish the offspring successfully. On the other hand there are clearly major cultural overlays which influence perception of body shape.

Sexual selection has also been suggested as one possible reason why humans have lost most of their body hair.

7.8   Gender differences in morbidity and mortality

In nearly all societies, women have a longer life expectancy than men (Figure 7.4). In developed countries, two-thirds of those over the age of 80 years are female. In part this difference is due to males being more vulnerable to extrinsic causes of death. Men are more likely to die of violence, and in the past from diseases related to smoking or alcohol consumption (although women have been catching up in this respect). In societies where violence is very much part of life, whether it be a war which can affect a generation, continual skirmishes with

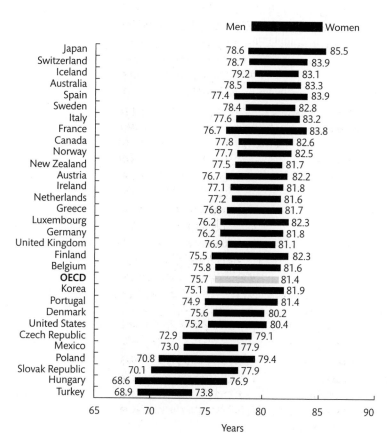

Figure 7.4 Women live longer than men in high-income countries. Figure shows life expectancy at birth of men and women. OECD, Organisation for Economic Co-operation and Development (modified from *Health at a Glance 2007: OECD Indicators* (2007), www.oecd.org/health/healthataglance, with permission).

neighbouring tribes, or in urban situations in which rival gangs fight over turf or two neighbours have a dispute, it is usually the males who fight and are killed. In many animal species the battle between rival males for reproductive supremacy is a constant feature of life. Males from the age of puberty are more likely to engage in risk-taking behaviour but males also have a higher intrinsic mortality rate. As shown in Figure 7.5, males are more likely to die at every age from birth. The male/female ratio in a Western society (USA) at birth to 10 years is 105%, at 50 years is 96%, and at 80 is 65%. The physiological reasons why males are more vulnerable to disease are complex and some non-human primates share this trend, but an evolutionary explanation is possible. Assuming humans evolved with a mildly polygynous mating system, then the female fitness strategy depends on a longer, healthier life, whereas males depend on a period of sexual dominance, which may be relatively transient, to maximize fitness.

An example of sexual dimorphism in disease risk is cardiovascular disease. Hypertension is a feature of younger men and post-menopausal women. Lifestyle, dietary, and exercise patterns do not explain this difference, and nor do patterns of smoking. It appears that oestrogens are protective and in women the disease process is enhanced by a reduction in oestrogen, leading to an increasing risk

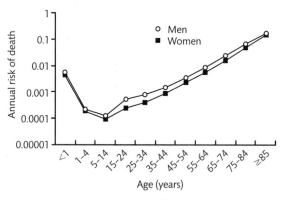

Figure 7.5 Risk of death by age and sex in a high-income country. At all ages, the risk of death is higher in men than in women; note in particular the divergence of the curves, disfavouring men, during the reproductive years of 15–44 years (data from *Mortality Statistics*, Series DH2 no. 32 (2006) Office for National Statistics, London).

after the menopause. Oestrogen acts via the oestrogen receptor α (ERα) on vasculature to enhance vasodilatation, which reduces remodelling of vascular smooth muscle and counteracts the effects of oxidative stress.

7.9 The human reproductive cycle

7.9.1 Puberty

Soon after birth, the fetal activation of the sex hormone system necessary for prenatal sexual differentiation (at least in the male) is suppressed by hypothalamic mechanisms. The precise nature of this 'gonadostat' is still uncertain but the hypothalamic–pituitary–gonadal axis then stays quiescent until puberty. In adrenarche, a poorly understood process that precedes puberty, the adrenal cortex markedly increases its production of adrenal androgens, starting in mid to late childhood (6–8 years). Adrenarche is generally covert but it can induce early and slight pubic hair production in both sexes. The function of adrenarche is unclear. But humans are distinct in having a pubertal growth spurt and in most other primates growth is largely complete by the age of sexual maturation. Thus adrenarche may in some way be an evolutionary echo of different controls on growth and maturation which operate across species (see Chapter 5).

At puberty, the gonadostat mechanism is reversed and gonadotrophin release is reactivated. This leads to the Leydig cells of the testis secreting testosterone and to the Sertoli cells supporting active spermatogenesis. In the female, ovarian follicles reactivate and start to secrete oestrogen and progesterone. Eventually this develops into a cyclical pattern due to changes in the feedback mechanism of oestradiol on luteinizing hormone release. Oestradiol generally acts as a negative-feedback controller of luteinizing hormone release, but in mid cycle it starts to exert positive feedback, leading to the pre-ovulatory luteinizing hormone surge and thus to ovulation. Follicular development recommences and the cyclical process, in which generally one oocyte fully matures and ovulates each cycle, is established.

Testosterone and oestrogens determine the development of secondary sexual characteristics. In males this causes pubic, facial, and axillary hair to develop, the larynx to change shape and shift its position downwards more surviving offspring can be enhanced if a woman stops having children in time to support the development of her youngest child. This may be a better strategy for a slow reproducing species to maximize fitness. It balances the cumulative and rising risk of death from the next pregnancy and childbirth against the survival of her last child which might otherwise perish if she dies. Thus in evolutionary terms it may pay to stop having children and to invest in those already born.

A second but non-mutually exclusive adaptive argument relies on the concept of inclusive fitness. A mother with many children may be limited in her capacity to support all of them. Thus as she ages her youngest may be compromised. But if she is helped by her own mother she can learn mothering skills at a younger age and more of her children are likely to survive. In turn, the grandmother assists her own fitness by ensuring more of her own children live until adulthood. This is the so-called **grandmother hypothesis**. Modelling again shows that it can confer a fitness advantage. It has empirical support in studies of child survival in Africa where child mortality is less in families where the maternal grandmother lives in the same village. The presence of the elder women and indeed older men might also confer other advantages through accumulated knowledge which can help a clan in times of stress. Analogous arguments have been used

to explain the role of the matriarch in an elephant herd. This might explain why human societies in general have maintained elderly people as an integral and respected component of the clan. Recent modelling studies suggest that a combination of these two adaptive arguments confers a greater fitness advantage (Box 7.6). Thus the consensus is that menopause is an evolved rather than an accidental phenomenon.

7.10 Conclusion: reproduction and evolution

Given that the net effect of evolutionary forces is eventually expressed through successful reproduction, it is to be expected that there is a broad diversity of reproductive strategies across the animal kingdom. This is a simple reflection of the diversity of biotic and abiotic environments that organisms have evolved to live within. Changes in reproductive strategy underlie, or are reflected in, key evolutionary steps such as the transition from unicellular to multicellular organisms. There is evidence from green algae species (*Volvox*) that cell differentiation into nutritionally supporting and reproductive cells was a key early component in the origin of complexity. The development of sexual reproduction appears to have had a major

---

Box 7.6   Using modelling studies to explain the menopause

Modelling can be a useful approach for investigating complex phenomena. It involves mathematical and computational analysis of theories for which parameters of known variables have been established. Modelling can then predict the outcomes when variables are changed.

The evolution of menopause in humans has been studied this way using survival and fecundity data on a Taiwanese pastoral population. To investigate the effects of human altriciality and grandmother assistance on the age of menopause, two models were generated to look at each factor in isolation, and a third model was developed to look at a composite of the two previous models. Many variables

were incorporated into the analyses, such as childbirth-induced maternal death, juvenile survival, fecundity, and availability of grandmother's assistance. Various combinations of the variables were examined under fixed or changing conditions. Essentially, it was shown that the first two models were insufficient to explain age at menopause. Only when the presence of the grandmother was combined with maternal survival for nurture of her youngest child did the model fit with available data. Indeed, this theoretical life history model was subsequently verified empirically using a comprehensive data set from The Gambia.

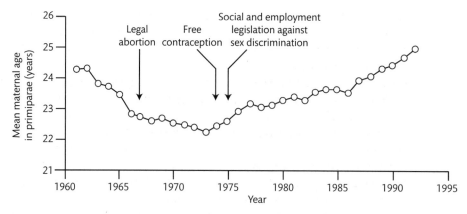

Figure 7.11 Secular trend in maternal age at first childbirth in the UK (modified from Glinianaia, S.V. *et al.* (2008) *BMC Pregnancy Childbirth* **8**, 39).

advantage in allowing organisms to survive in complex biotic environments and to sustain defences against parasites. Placentation emerged several times across taxa, and combined with lactation has created the basic mammalian reproductive strategy. It requires considerable pre- and postnatal maternal investment, which in turn creates a number of gender-related interactions. The evolution of mammalian imprinting appears to be directly linked to the evolution of therian (placental) mammals.

The human life history has a number of distinct elements. These include delayed maturation, single fetuses, a long inter-birth interval, high post-partum parental investment and, in females, complete reproductive decline before the end of the lifespan, at least in the modern world. Both the social and physical environment prior to maturity can affect age at puberty. The changing relationship between the age of physical maturation and the age of acceptance or performance as an adult in developed societies have consequences for mental and societal health. Equally, the rapid change in female reproductive behaviour associated with women's empowerment and widespread use of effective contraception has led to a major change in when women choose to have their first child (Figure 7.11). This changing reproductive behaviour is in conflict with our evolved biology, by which ovarian function declines from the age of about 35. This mismatch between expectation and biology is partially addressed through assisted reproductive technology such as *in vitro* fertilization.

KEY POINTS

- Sexual reproduction is not universal and the favoured hypothesis is that it evolved as a strategy to address the threat of parasites.

- There is a broad range of reproductive strategies across species, which have evolved to maximize fitness for each species and each sex according to the physical, biotic, and social environments.

- The investment of males and females in reproduction is very different. Each species has evolved strategies in which an equilibrium of interests between the sexes is reached. This is reflected in patterns of parental investment, mate choice, and social structure.

- The mammalian reproductive strategy relies on placentation and lactation to provide nutritional support and immune and physical protection to the offspring.

- The human reproductive strategy includes a delayed puberty and few generally singleton pregnancies with a high parental investment in the offspring.

- The timing of puberty is influenced by developmental influences, and there is a potential disconnection between the age of biological puberty and acceptance as an adult; this is reflected in the problems of adolescence.

humans reach their lowest level of body fat in the life cycle (see Chapter 5). If the threat of famine is what drove the human tendency to build up fat reserves, it is not obvious why children's bodies should do so little to prepare for these difficult periods. The lower priority placed upon maintaining an energy reserve by middle childhood suggests that the background risk of starvation faced by our ancestors – 'famine' – was small in comparison to the nutritional stress during the preceding developmental

period of infancy. Indeed, infancy is marked by often intensive nutritional stress associated with weaning and the related problem of infectious disease, making nutritional disruption and nutrition-related mortality common at this age (see Box 8.8). Because all individuals who successfully pass on their genes to offspring must have survived this early-life nutritional bottleneck, there is likely to have been selection for building up protective fat reserves at this age in large-brained humans.

Box 8.8 Why are human babies fat?

Humans have been described as naturally obese, a characterization which is particularly apt at birth as humans are born with more body fat than any other species (Figure 8.6). Attempts to explain our unusual 'baby fat' traditionally looked to our hairlessness for clues, and it was assumed that natural selection compensated for our loss of fur with a layer of insulative blubber. A newer perspective notes that this excess adipose tissue is well suited to serve as a back-up energy supply for another distinctive human trait: our large brains. Brains have among the highest metabolic rates of any tissue or organ in the body, and they are quickly damaged in the event of even temporary disruption in energy

supply. Humans are exceptional in the size of our brains, especially early in life, and roughly 70–80% of the body's metabolism is devoted to this costly organ in the newborn (see Chapter 5).

Although brains are clearly critical to our social and cognitive capacities, having a large brain poses a special metabolic challenge to a newborn. First, they increase energy requirements above what would be expected for the young of a smaller-brained species. Second, unlike energy expended on other tissues or systems, brain metabolism may not be reduced to conserve energy during a crisis, but must be maintained within narrow limits to avoid permanent damage. Thus, our large brains impose a

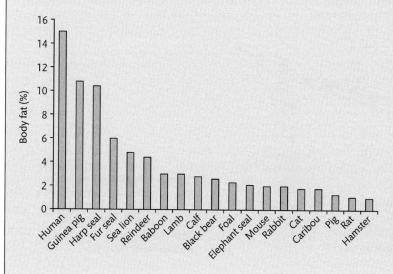

Figure 8.6 Humans are born fat: percentage body fat at birth in mammals (modified from Kuzawa, C.W. (1998) *American Journal of Physical Anthropology* **Suppl. 27,** 177–209, with permission).

double burden on metabolism during infancy: they increase energy demands while restricting flexibility in expenditure when nutritional supply is disrupted.

Other factors that are commonly experienced during infancy can impede the supply of nutrients, ensuring that negative energy balance is a frequent occurrence at this age across most populations. We are born with a naïve adaptive immune system, and must therefore come into contact with (and be infected by) specific pathogens to acquire the repertoire of antibodies necessary to protect us from future infection. Breastfed infants are initially shielded from pathogens, and are often quite healthy in the early postnatal months. But as energy requirements outstrip the supply of breast milk by roughly 6 months of age (Figure 8.7), less sterile complementary foods must be introduced, and infectious disease becomes unavoidable in all but the most sanitary settings. These childhood infections, in turn, are a source of nutritional stress, and indeed it is primarily through their effects on nutritional status that they compromise health and contribute to mortality during infancy and childhood. Once sick, a child loses appetite and this is often compounded by the withholding of food by caretakers. The common diarrhoeal diseases reduce

nutrient absorption and digestion, while the fevers associated with many viral infections can increase metabolic rate and thus energy expenditure. While the specific symptoms vary by illness, the ensuing nutritional depletion has the effect of suppressing immune function, leaving the infant more prone to future infection and a compounding cycle of nutritional stress.

The human infant thus faces a profound energetic dilemma: at precisely the age when they are most dependent upon caretaker provisioning to maintain the high and obligatory energy needs of their large brains, they are most likely to be cut off from that supply chain as a result of illness and the nutritional stresses of weaning. It is this confluence of factors, and the synergy between nutritional stress and compromised immunity, that accounts for much of the high infant mortality in many societies. In light of these risks, natural selection probably favoured neonatal adiposity as a strategy to prepare for this difficult period. It is not difficult to imagine how infants who deposit copious quantities of energy as fat prior to weaning would be better represented among the subset who survive to adulthood to reproduce and pass on their genes. It is also important to note that these sources of energy stress have largely receded

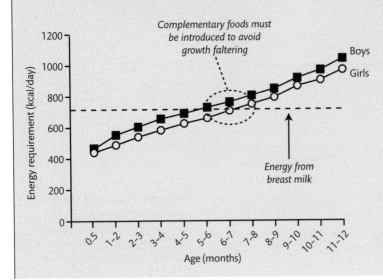

Figure 8.7 Breast feeding must be supplemented with complementary foods by around the sixth month of life to avoid growth faltering (figure courtesy of Dr Chris Kuzawa, Northwestern University).

correlation between rates of neonatal mortality (a marker of poverty, and indirectly of maternal nutrition) in the 1920s and rates of death from coronary heart disease several decades later.

What might account for such an association between early-life and late-life mortality? These observations were very remote in time, and likely to be influenced by unmeasured factors, such as differences in smoking, diet, or lifestyle, which were not quantifiable. The next step was to move from gross correlations over integrated populations and across time to find out what happened to a specific population where individuals could be studied throughout their lives. What was needed was a set of records about the growth and development of children in the early part of the century that could be linked specifically to the causes of death in later life. With the assistance of an archivist, Barker and his colleagues scoured Britain for records about birth and infancy dating from the early part of the century. They of course found many such records, but most were incomplete or scanty in detail and many had been stored in poor conditions where they had deteriorated.

The largest set of records which were found related to the English county of Hertfordshire. These included weight at birth, weight at 1 year of age, and whether the baby was weaned at 1 year. The ledgers

had been maintained from 1911 to 1945. Barker and his colleagues used the National Health Service Central Register at Southport to trace 16 000 men and women born in Hertfordshire between 1911 and 1930, and to determine their cause of death. The results – first published in 1989 – were controversial. What they found, for both men and women, was that risk of death from heart disease was doubled in individuals born with a weight of less than 5.5 lbs compared to those born with a weight of more than 9.5 lbs.

Other workers also showed that excess nutrition in infancy, such as associated with formula feeding, also led to altered disease risk. Given that poor fetal growth is generally associated with some rebound rapid infant growth these are probably different perspectives on the same phenomenon. However, further evaluation of the developmental data showed that the relationship between developmental growth patterns and disease risk is not a function of severe intra-uterine growth impairment; rather, there is a continuous change in risk across the full range of developmental growth patterns (Figure 8.10). This suggests that disease risk is not a consequence of developmental disruption but is part of a developmentally plastic process that originally had adaptive purpose.

evidence from modern famines (see Box 8.11) further supports the role of the intra-uterine environment in determining health in later life.

8.6.1 Maladaptive consequences of an adaptive process

The retrospective epidemiological studies could not provide evidence about the biological basis of the relationship, but a consensus arose that a poor fetal or early-life experience altered development in such a way that growth was affected and also influenced the propensity to develop disease in latter life. The term programming, previously used to reflect the later consequences of formula

versus breastfeeding or early environmental influences on sexual differentiation, was adopted to describe the phenomenon. Subsequently, Barker and Hales developed the **thrifty phenotype hypothesis**, an explicit reference to Neel's earlier proposal of a thrifty genotype, to explain programming. Their concept was that the fetus adjusts its biology in response to signals from its mother of poor nutrition, allowing it to survive until birth but predisposing it to the adverse consequences of such programmed thriftiness in adulthood.

Animal studies have been used to confirm and extend the results from humans and dissect the underlying molecular mechanisms. The initial studies were performed in rats. If a rat fetus was undernourished *in utero*,

Box 8.11   Modern famines

The improvement in farming efficiency in the twentieth century arising from mechanization and use of chemical fertilizers has not ended famine. Indeed, some commentators claim that even the great famines of history were never the result of food shortages alone but always had some exacerbating sociopolitical dimension. Such claims are supported by examination of the factors precipitating some of the famines of the last century, such as the Ukrainian famine of the 1930s in the Soviet Union associated with forced collectivization, the disastrous famine in China that followed Mao's Great Leap Forward in the 1950s, and the association of famine with political instability in the Horn of Africa that continues to this day.

Medicine contributes to alleviation of the effects of famine, but famine sadly provides scientists with an opportunity to examine one extreme of human nutritional physiology. Such natural experiments build our knowledge of how undernutrition during pregnancy affects the growth and later health of the offspring, but the social disruption that accompanies famine usually means that medical records and the opportunity for follow-up of affected individuals are lost, and famine is usually protracted, so that separation of effects on gestation from those on infant and childhood nutrition is difficult. Few famines are temporally circumscribed events during which adequate social and medical records are kept, but some are, and several cohort studies exist of twentieth-century populations whose nutrition was affected by armed conflict. Such cohorts include those from the Spanish Civil War of 1936–1939, the siege of Leningrad from 1941 to 1944, and the Dutch Hunger Winter of 1944–1945.

The rapid advance of Allied troops across Western Europe after the Normandy invasion in June 1944 was halted in September by the failure of the operation to seize the 'bridge too far' across the Rhine at Arnhem in the Netherlands. Reprisals on the Dutch civilian population for their cooperation with the Allies, followed by a severe winter, meant that food and fuel supplies in the western cities of the Netherlands were extremely limited between November 1944 and the liberation of the country in May 1945. Although the population was relatively well nourished before this period of famine, and food supplies were restored quickly after liberation, energy intake during the peak months of deprivation was no more than 400–800 calories per day. In spite of these difficulties, medical care for pregnant women continued and detailed records of their food intake, the course of their pregnancies, and their babies' size at birth were maintained. The availability of these records has allowed the lifelong health of the children of the Hunger Winter, who are now in late middle age, to be correlated with their exposure to undernutrition *in utero* at various stages of gestation and compared with that of a control group of people from the same area who were born in the months before, or conceived in the months after, the famine.

Only exposure to famine in late gestation had marked effect on birth size, with both length and weight being reduced. As might be expected from the epidemiological studies of Barker and colleagues described in Box 8.10, babies born small because of third-trimester maternal undernutrition developed glucose intolerance and high blood pressure in later life. But even though exposure to famine in early or middle gestation had no effect on birth size, such babies also showed markers of ill-health as adults, including glucose intolerance, altered blood lipid profiles and blood coagulation, and increased stress sensitivity. These abnormalities were associated with an increased risk of coronary heart disease. In addition, women exposed to famine in their early gestation were more obese as adults than unexposed women and had a markedly higher risk of developing breast cancer.

because the pregnant dam was fed a reduced-energy diet or just an unbalanced diet (e.g. low protein content), it became hypertensive as an adult. These adult rats were also shown to have insulin resistance and to have shorter life expectancies than those whose mothers had been fed a balanced diet in pregnancy. The effect was magnified if the rat was placed on a high-fat diet after weaning, echoing the human situation of dietary abundance and demonstrating that the interaction between the fetal and postnatal environments determined outcome. Indeed, there are compelling data that excess nutrition in the young infant independent of fetal experience leads to an increased disease risk, and formula feeding provides much more energy than human milk to the infant.

As experimental work proceeded it became linked to other fields of biological enquiry, especially evolutionary developmental biology (see Chapter 4). The realization was growing that development was an important and under-represented component. But a key feature of the link with metabolic disease was that this was not just about those with low birthweight. The epidemiological studies had shown a continuous relationship between birth size and latter disease risk, present even in those of above average birth size (Figure 8.10). Experimentalists had also shown that metabolic programming could be induced by changes in the fetal environment which did not affect birthweight. Further epidemiological and

clinical studies showed that smaller infants had relatively more visceral fat (see Box 8.1) at birth, although subcutaneous fat was reduced, and that those who ended up developing diabetes had a different pattern of fat development from infancy (Figure 8.11). Such observations, together with the broad incidence of metabolic disease in the population, suggested that the developmental component did not represent the outcome of a pathological process where fetal development was disrupted. It was rather a maladaptive outcome of the generally adaptive processes of developmental plasticity. Indeed, there is evidence that lifelong epigenetic changes in genes associated with systems such as insulin sensitivity, glucose metabolism, and the glucocorticoid axis underpin the developmental induction of metabolic risk.

8.6.2 Developmental plasticity in the setting of evolutionary novelty

How can these developmental components be understood in evolutionary terms: is a synthesis between the evolutionary novelty and developmental concepts possible? For instance, why might birthweight relate inversely to risk for later metabolic disease, not just at the extremes of lowest birthweight, but across most of the entire birthweight distribution? (Very large babies are often born to mothers with gestational diabetes, and these babies are also at risk via a

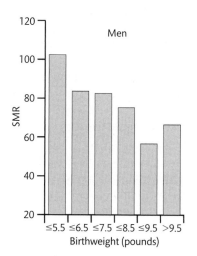
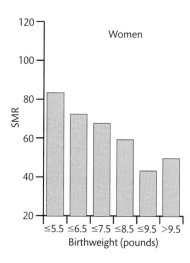

Figure 8.10 The relationship between birthweight and death from coronary heart disease (expressed as standardized mortality ratio, SMR) is continuous across the range of birthweights (modified from Godfrey, K. (2006) in *Developmental Origins of Health and Disease* (Gluckman, P.D. & Hanson, M., eds), Cambridge University Press, Cambridge with permission).

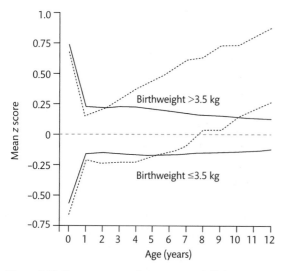

Figure 8.11 Two separate pathways to type 2 diabetes: low birthweight followed by catch-up growth, or high birthweight followed by accelerated weight gain through childhood. Lines represent trajectories of body weight difference from cohort mean (z score); broken lines represent those who were destined to develop diabetes (from Eriksson, J. *et al.* (2003) *Diabetes Care* **26**, 3006–3010, with permission).

different pathway: see section 8.6.3.) As discussed above, this suggests that these processes are not pathological in origin but are fundamental to biological variation operating in the normal range. Chapter 4 detailed how the processes of developmental plasticity act to allow one genotype to give rise to a range of phenotypes and how organisms use plasticity as an alternative or additional process to adapt to environments, particularly among species faced with change during their life course. Developmentally plastic responses are induced by external cues, and depending on the fidelity of the relationship between the cue and the future environment, there may be effects on fitness or health.

It was hypothesized that if the developing organism predicts a future limited nutritional environment, it might be appropriate to use the mechanisms of plasticity to adjust growth patterns so that later body function is optimized for a limiting nutritional environment. Conversely, if the fetus predicts a later nutritionally luxurious environment, it is appropriate to have metabolic systems set up with different expectations. In the former situation of predicted nutritional threat, an appropriate

response would include reduced investment in somatic growth (e.g. reduced muscle mass), a preference for high-fat foods, metabolic settings that favour fat deposition in times of energy excess, and altered endocrine, behavioural, and vascular controls such that the organism has reduced insulin secretion and sensitivity (Figure 8.12). Given that evolution is driven by the fitness imperative, anticipation of a threatening environment might be expected to accelerate the timing of maturation and commit more resources to reproduction, perhaps even at a cost to other traits that improve longevity (for instance, by investing less in cellular or DNA repair).

The adaptive advantage of a predictive response would depend on the fidelity of the prediction. If correct predictions lead to greater chances of growth and survival to reproduce, this would be why underlying anticipatory processes have been selected through evolution. When fetal nutrition is not a reliable cue of external conditions, as a result of maternal disease, placental inadequacy or malfunction, or simply because the environment has changed notably between birth and later life, this could produce a phenotype not well suited to meeting the challenges of its environment and thus at greater risk of disease. In the metabolic domain, a phenotype of increased insulin resistance, reduced muscle mass, and increased propensity to store fat is precisely the background on which susceptibility to metabolic disease would be enhanced in a later nutritional environment of high energy availability.

The developmental mismatch model proposes that in evolutionary terms there is an advantage in using the processes of developmental plasticity to adjust the set points for metabolic homeostasis to match the predicted mature environment. This process could have had adaptive advantage in environments that were reasonably stable over decades. But the fidelity of the prediction might increasingly be lost because the mechanisms of maternal constraint (see Box 8.13) limit the forecast that is possible, particularly as the postnatal environment grows abundant in evolutionarily unprecedented ways. Additionally, modern lifeways allow a greater range of fetuses to survive, many with greater degrees of maternal constraint (such as twins and those with extreme growth retardation) and perhaps therefore with a greater risk of mismatch. Maternal ill-health and placental dysfunction are other ways in which the maternal–placental transduction of

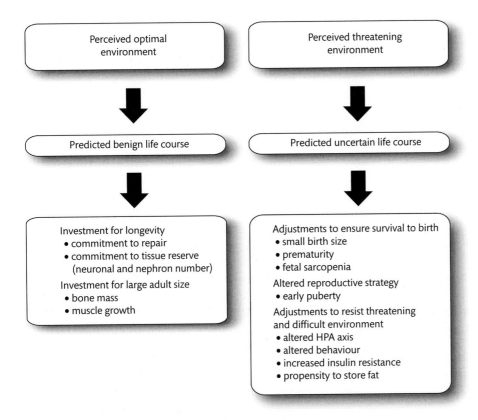

Figure 8.12 Integrated life history responses to developmental cues: examples of developmental trajectories in response to predicted adequate or deprived nutritional environments. HPA axis, hypothalamic–pituitary–gonadal axis (modified from Gluckman, P. *et al.* (2007) *American Journal of Human Biology* **19**, 1–19, with permission).

environmental information can lead to a faulty prediction and progress in obstetrics and paediatrics allow a far greater range of babies to survive to adulthood.

While the expansion of experimental and clinical research and the definition of underlying epigenetic mechanisms has established the view that developmental pathways are important, the relative importance of these pathways in contributing to risk of metabolic disease remains uncertain. Clearly disease risk would not exist were it not for the large change in diet and lifestyle discussed in previous sections. The point that emerges from this discussion is that developmental factors *per se* do not cause obesity or insulin resistance; rather, depending on the developmental trajectory induced early in life, the individual is more or less likely to develop insulin resistance and metabolic compromise in an obesogenic environment.

8.6.3 Other possible developmental pathways

There are other developmental pathways to obesity which also have an element of novelty. Women who have gestational diabetes give birth to babies with greater fat mass. High maternal glucose levels lead to high fetal glucose levels as placental glucose transfer is partially concentration-dependent. This leads to a rise in fetal insulin release and high fetal insulin levels lead to excess fetal adipogenesis. As fat cell number is primarily determined in fetal life, having more fat cells makes these individuals more likely to get fat in later life in a modern environment, and in turn to develop insulin resistance and type 2 diabetes. In a sense this can also be considered evolutionarily novel in that this is a pathological pathway: gestational diabetes is likely to be primarily a recent phenomenon associated with the nutritional transition and medical advances.

Box 8.12   Reversal of developmental metabolic effects

A person's susceptibility to metabolic disease in later life is partly determined by events that occur before birth, but birthweight alone is not a reliable marker for such programming. Tests to predict when programming has occurred, and the availability of interventions to reverse programming could reduce the prevalence of adult-onset chronic disease. There is growing evidence for the role of epigenetic processes in developmental plasticity and it is likely that epigenetic control of expression of a few key genes is responsible for the alterations of metabolic set points that predispose a person to develop obesity or diabetes. High-throughput methods to assess epigenetic change are now becoming available, and if key regulatory genes can be identified then measurement of their epigenetic status in tissues easily available at birth (such as umbilical cord blood) could be used to predict a person's future susceptibility to disease.

But what could be done when increased risk is predicted? If susceptibility to obesity and diabetes is identified at birth, then parents and later the individual could be advised about dietary modification to reduce the risk. Neonatal testing and dietary intervention is effective for some monogenic disorders of metabolism such as phenylketonuria,

whose devastating nature encourages compliance (see Chapter 3). But experience shows that lifestyle interventions for the chronic adult-onset diseases are much less effective. Wouldn't it be better in this case to reverse the programming process? Recent work suggests that this might in fact be possible.

When rats are undernourished during pregnancy, their pups are born small and thin but grow up to be lethargic, gluttonous, and obese, with changes in metabolic parameters similar to those seen in human type 2 diabetes; this is especially true if they are fed a high-fat diet after weaning. But if these 'programmed' rats are treated for a short period after birth with injections of the adipokine leptin, all the deleterious changes in the adult animals are prevented. Leptin is produced by fat cells as a signal of adiposity, and it is likely that exposure to high levels of leptin early in life 'tricked' the animals into believing that they were fat and caused them to adjust their metabolic set points accordingly (leptin administration in the neonatal rat has marked effects on hypothalamic organization). Moreover, the adult 'couch potato' animals showed changes in expression and epigenetic status of key metabolic genes, and these changes were reversed by the leptin treatment.

Obese women give birth to babies with increased fat cell mass who are thus prone to become obese in an energy-dense environment. The mechanism is uncertain, but presumably there is excess nutrient transfer across the placenta which is incorporated into fat. Recent data show that infants who are breastfed have a lower incidence of obesity that those who are formula-fed. Bottle feeding is itself an evolutionary novelty and may be providing high levels of particular nutrients that have a compromising

effect or induce epigenetic change, or it might simply be that the higher energy content of cows' milk over human milk exacerbates mismatch.

8.7   Conclusion

This chapter has demonstrated how an evolutionary perspective provides a clearer insight into the epidemic of

---

> **Box 8.13** **Could our upright posture have a role in the propensity to metabolic disease?**
>
> The importance of fetal nutrition as an influence on long-term risk for metabolic disease raises intriguing possibilities about the factors influencing adult health. Human fetal nutrition is under unique constraints owing to our large brain size at birth and the change in pelvic shape associated with the adoption of bipedalism. This reorientation required the evolution of mechanisms to closely match fetal size with the size of the pelvic opening, both of which vary across women. What this means is that it would be risky for fetal growth to be primarily determined by genetic factors. Mating of a small mother to a larger male, a presumably common feature in any sexually dimorphic species, leads to the risk of fetal overgrowth which would be fatal to both mother and infant and potentially to the species. Thus mechanisms exist to limit fetal growth to match maternal size. This can be demonstrated in embryo-transfer experiments and cross-breeding experiments in animals and by observations showing that, in the offspring of pregnancies in which ovum donation has been made, birth size is more closely correlated with recipient-mother size than donor-mother size. The mechanisms of such maternal constraint are poorly understood, but are likely to involve limitation of nutrient transfer to the fetus (see also Chapter 7).
>
> The degree of maternal constraint is not constant; it is greater in first-borns who are born smaller (and have a greater consequential risk of obesity). Constraint is greater in multiple pregnancies and is of particular relevance in shorter mothers, explaining the relationship between maternal height and birth size. Thus, in historical terms, women in a place like India, whose height is approximately 155 cm compared to 170 cm in Western women, give birth to smaller babies (2.7 compared with 3.5 kg) and this greater maternal constraint would lead to potentially greater risk of postnatal mismatch. It has been argued that this may go some way towards explaining why South Asian people tend to be at higher risk of metabolic disease at a lower level of obesity.
>
> It is proposed that in evolutionary terms this was not problematic: it did not compromise genetic fitness as the degree of maternal constraint was roughly matched with the energy/nutritional environment of the pre-agricultural human, where the postnatal diet was also generally limiting rather than excessive. But such a model could explain why even in a generalist species such as *Homo sapiens* there is an absolute limit on the nutritional environment we can adapt to and live in healthily. There is a limit on the environments a fetus can predict postnatally and thus predictively adapt to. This speculative paradigm provides a developmental source of individual variation in sensitivity beyond a purely genomic explanation.

metabolic diseases such as obesity and type 2 diabetes. It is the body's limited capacity to adapt to changing environments that ultimately lies at the heart of these diseases.

Members of a species gradually adapt to their nutritional environment through natural selection operating on genes which regulate metabolism and thus influence how the body manages its finite energy supply and expenditure. This process of genetic adaptation is slow but powerful, and through time members of a species come to have metabolic machineries well suited to the conditions that they routinely experience. New evidence is revealing how we also have a capacity to adjust our metabolic priorities developmentally in response to conditions and cues experienced early in life, beginning *in utero*. That is, our bodies appear to have the ability to 'learn' about local nutrition, not unlike the way we learn languages or other skills. Together, these two modes of adaptation allow organisms to cope with long-term and gradual changes and with more fine-grained changes that occur across decades or generations.

Despite the best efforts of these mechanisms, rapid environmental change can outstrip their ability to accommodate it. Metabolic diseases can be understood as a symptom of the resultant mismatch between an organism's biology and its environment. When environmental change is rapid relative to the rate of natural selection, the consequent gene–environment mismatch will drive disease. We have abundant evidence, albeit mostly indirect, that this is an important influence on human health. The human genome was selected over millions of years for a lifestyle of foraging and continues to 'expect' a diet high in protein, low in fat, and free from novelties such as refined sugars. Even if the search for specific metabolic disease-related genes has posed challenges, it seems undeniable that the bulk of the world's ballooning waistlines reflect patterns of cultural and dietary change coming into conflict with an increasingly obsolete genotype.

But mismatch between genes and environments may only be part of the story, for there is also evidence that an individual's early-life nutritional experiences influence how the body handles nutrition later in life, suggesting that when the pace of change is particularly rapid within a single lifetime or between generations, the body's capacity to adjust developmental biology in response to early nutrition can lead to a different form of mismatch: that between the biological settings established early in life and the nutritional and lifestyle conditions experienced subsequently.

This chapter has shown how both concurrent and developmental mismatch could work together to drive the modern global epidemic of metabolic diseases: gene–environment mismatch resulting from historically recent changes in diet and physical activity is largely responsible for the rise of conditions like obesity as a global phenomenon. As populations experience dietary change and gain weight, the impact on health depends upon that population's recent nutritional history. Populations with a high prevalence of individuals in the developing world who were born as lower-birthweight babies, for example as a result of maternal stunting, will be worse

---

KEY POINTS

- The bulk of human evolution occurred in a very different nutritional milieu and the human genotype was selected to be well adapted to that milieu.

- There is a rising incidence of obesity and its associated disorders in both the developed and developing worlds.

- There has been a rapid change in diet and behaviour against the background of a genotype that cannot change rapidly.

- Developmental processes may also contribute to the rising incidence of metabolic mismatch.

---

off as they gain weight. Maternal obesity and gestational diabetes exacerbate the transmission of risk to the next generation. Such models can help explain differences in disease susceptibility in populations at different points in the nutrition transition or experiencing change at different rates. In all cases, it is adaptability – or, more precisely, the limits of adaptability – that lies at the heart of this modern global scourge.

Further reading

Barker, D.J.P. (1998) *Mothers, Babies and Health in Later Life*, 2nd edn. Churchill Livingstone, Edinburgh.

Cohen, M.N. and Armelagos, G.J. (eds) (1984) *Paleopathology at the Origins of Agriculture*. Academic Press, New York.

Coll, A.P., Farooqi, I.S., and O'Rahilly, S. (2007) The hormonal control of food intake. *Cell* **129**, 251–262.

Eaton, S.B., Shostack, M., and Konner, M. (1988) *The Paleolithic Prescription*. Harper and Row, New York.

Fogel, R.W. (2004) *The Escape from Hunger and Premature Death, 1700–2100: Europe, America and the Third World*. Cambridge University Press, Cambridge.

Gluckman, P.D. and Hanson, M.A. (eds) (2006) *Developmental Origins of Health and Disease*. Cambridge University Press, Cambridge.

Box 9.5 Breast versus bottle feeding

Current guidelines recommend exclusive breast-feeding for the first 6 months of infancy. Breast milk provides all the nutrients required at this age in a form that is hygienic and easy to digest. The protein, carbohydrate, and fat profiles are unique to breast milk and differ in many ways from those in the milk from other animals such as cows. Breast milk also contains a range of bioactive components, including antimicrobial and anti-inflammatory factors, digestive enzymes, hormones, and growth factors. Antimicrobial agents include leucocytes, secretory immunoglobulin (Ig) A, IgM, and IgG antibodies, oligosaccharides, lysozyme, lactoferrin, complement, lipids, fatty acids, and mucins. Growth factors such as insulin-like growth factor 1 (IGF-1) and epidermal growth factor (EGF) are thought to be important for gut maturation. Lactoferrin is one of several specific binders in human milk which greatly increase the bioavailability of micronutrients.

Breastfeeding is a life-saver for children in developing countries, where sterile water and bottles may not be available. There have been many tragic cases of death from infant diarrhoea as a result of the feeding of formula aggressively marketed by food companies in conditions where it could not be properly prepared. There are many beneficial effects of breastfeeding on all children. They include: reduced risk of infection, especially of the gastrointestinal tract, lung, and ear; more appropriate growth patterns, with lower risk of childhood obesity; reduced risk of type 2 diabetes and cardiovascular disease; better cognitive function and neurodevelopment; reduced incidence of allergy and atopic disease; improved bone health; and a reduced risk of breast cancer in the mothers.

Despite these obvious benefits not all women can or do breastfeed their infants for the 6-month period recommended. Cultural attitudes to breastfeeding and the lack of appropriate facilities in the workplace contribute to this, and social class and education play a major role.

---

strains of commensals in the mother and her offspring. These commensals may be transferred during birth, and this can be considered a further form of non-genomic inheritance.

On the other hand, some gut biota use the human gut as a parasitic host environment. Tapeworms, trematodes (flatworms or flukes), and roundworms passage their eggs/larvae to other hosts through human faeces. Some infestation is direct, via water or vegetation contamination; sometimes it involves an intermediate host, for example the water snail in bilharzia. These parasites compete for nutrients with human absorption and can cause considerable malnutrition with long-term consequences as well as abdominal distress for many, particularly in the developing world.

9.3.2 Pathogen emergence

There are over 1200 species of recognized human pathogen, although the majority of infection-related mortality and morbidity is caused by just a few of these: malaria, HIV/AIDS, and tuberculosis. This multiplicity of threats imposes a continual interplay between our defence systems and the transmissability and virulence of these organisms. Many pathogens, including viruses, some bacteria (some species of *Chlamydia*), and some parasites (for example, malaria and *Leishmania*) require the human as a host to allow for their own survival and reproduction.

To be a pathogen, an organism must be able to survive in and replicate in its host, and must be transmissible between hosts (sometimes via an intermediate vector). Microbial fitness is often expressed as basic reproductive rate, R_0, the average number of progeny produced. R_0 must be greater than 1 if a micro-organism is to persist within its host population, whereas host defences operate to drive R_0 below 1 so that the infection will die out. By definition, a pathogen must negatively affect the host organism; it may do this by secreting a toxin, damaging cellular function, competing for nutrients, or simply by causing mechanical damage.

Patterns of pathogen-induced disease are not the same across the globe. Environmental factors play a part in this; for example, the conditions suitable for mosquitoes to breed are confined to tropical and subtropical climates with pools of water. Historically, malaria was endemic in southern Europe well into the twentieth century, and climate change may mean that the disease may well become widespread there again. However, historical considerations reveal that there may be more to explaining patterns of disease. Why, for example, do the diseases of the tropics include chronic infections and infestations such as bilharzia and onchocerciasis and those of more temperate regions include infections such as smallpox and tuberculosis? One hypothesis is that the tropical pattern emerged through co-evolution of the responsible pathogens in consort with ancestral hominids in Africa. Low population density and nomadic lifestyle may have favoured the evolution of chronic diseases with relatively low virulence and the need for intermediate vectors such as the mosquito, tsetse fly, and water snail. The more recent migration into temperate regions was accompanied by the development of settlements with higher population density and the development of animal husbandry, favouring diseases with a zoonotic origin, or with higher virulence and more direct person-to-person transmission. In addition to the adoption of a sedentary lifestyle, temperate-zone hominids began to domesticate animals. Living in closer proximity with such animals favoured the transmission of pathogens from them to humans, and this may be the origin of diseases such as tuberculosis.

But what determines the transmission of an infectious disease from animals to humans? Why is it a relatively rare event? The answer seems to be that the successful shift in host from animal to human involves several distinct events. Consider the influenza A virus H5N1, a strain of avian influenza which has only infected a few humans who have been in particularly close contact with handling raw chicken meat, but about which there is much concern for the potential for human-to-human transmission. Studies of the influenza pandemics of 1918, 1957, and 1968 give some clues. Influenza viruses are endemic in bird populations, both in the wild and in domesticated species, and in some other animals such as pigs, and they are highly mutable. Each pandemic is thought to represent the emergence of mutated forms that have

escaped the immunity of previous influenza infections in humans and successfully made the transition from reproducing in an animal host to reproducing in a human host. The so-called Spanish flu virus which produced the 1918 pandemic in which 50 million people died worldwide appears to have been due to the transfer of a complete avian virus into humans. In contrast, the more common influenza A virus shows a relatively linear evolution. The antigenic properties of the influenza virus change from year to year as a result of mutation (antigenic drift), necessitating the production of new vaccines and annual vaccination of susceptible members of the population. But on top of this there have been several large shifts in antigenicity in the past century ('Asian flu' in 1957; 'Hong Kong flu' in 1968) arising from reassortment of genes between two viral strains co-infecting an individual. Close proximity between humans and animal hosts offers the potential for initial direct inoculation (for instance, through a cut). In the case of H5N1, the first transmission to humans was reported in 1997 and this is the stage at which H5N1 currently exists: infection from the animal host can occur, but human-to-human transmission remains unconfirmed. The critical next step will be if the H5N1 virus exchanges genomic material with a flu virus that has the potential to be transmitted between humans because it can bind to surface receptors on cells in the human respiratory tract. If this happens a pandemic could result, because there may be little resistance in the human population in any country. Given that viruses replicate with very short generation times, the chance of individual mutations are high. The cumulative effect of those mutations in inducing a virulent pathogen depends on whether the human defence mechanisms are adequate or whether technology in the form of isolation, vaccination, or medication can reduce the spread of the organism and contain the epidemic.

9.3.3 Virulence

Whether or not we succumb to an infection is often not much a question of whether we have come into contact with the pathogen, but rather the size of the infectious load and the virulence of the particular strain. Simple procedures such as hand-washing greatly reduce the risk of cross-infections in hospitals by reducing the exposure load; the major advance in patient survival after surgery afforded by the invention of the crude but effective carbolic acid spray by Lister in 1869 was due to the reduction of bacterial load rather than achieving complete sterility, a principle that stills holds true today in operating theatres.

Organisms may have very different virulence. At its simplest, virulence is the measure of an infecting organism's ability to cause morbidity and mortality in its host. Virulence may appear as incidental damage to the host that does not benefit the infecting organism or as damage that does benefit the infecting organism (most commonly, by enhancing its transmission). For example, the principal morbidity caused by HIV is gradual destruction of the host's immune system, increasing susceptibility to opportunistic infections and malignancy. This type of damage to the host does not benefit the virus by enhancing its (mostly) sexual transmission, although the temporal pattern of the infection, with a long asymptomatic period during which numerous sexual partners can be infected, does promote transmission. Contrast this with cholera, ingested perhaps via water contaminated with faeces containing the bacterium. The organism clings to the wall of the gut and secretes a toxin which triggers the secretion of serous fluid and this rapidly produces violent diarrhoea. This trait is adaptive for the *Vibrio* organism in that it allows greater spread to other hosts. We might predict that selection on the infecting organism will act to optimize net transmission between hosts, trading off high virulence (high transmission, but killing the host quickly) against low virulence (low transmission, but the host survives long enough to infect multiple other hosts). Optimizing this trade-off will be particularly important for sexually transmitted infections, since high morbidity will reduce mating opportunities. We should also remember that the host response can contribute to virulence: the case fatality rate in the 1918 Spanish flu pandemic was particularly high because the virus elicited an aberrant host immune response that caused extensive tissue damage in the lungs, which may explain its unusual pattern of age-specific mortality (Figure 9.2).

Returning to the example of cholera, different strains have evolved different virulence in accordance with their relationship to the host. A high level of virulence will generate a high degree of fluid secretion into the gut and the bacteria will be quickly washed out, speeding their transmission. On the other hand, the production of toxin carries a metabolic cost and so this has to be traded-off against the fitness benefits of rapid transmission. But very highly virulent organisms that are newly infecting humans, such as Ebola and avian influenza, both of which have high case fatality rates, may be easier to contain because where rates of mortality are high and incubation times are low, the organism's ability to spread to a large number of hosts may be limited. Isolation and quarantine effectively achieve the same outcome, of limiting the host pool.

Virulence is also affected by the host's biology and behaviour. Consider typhoid fever, caused by the

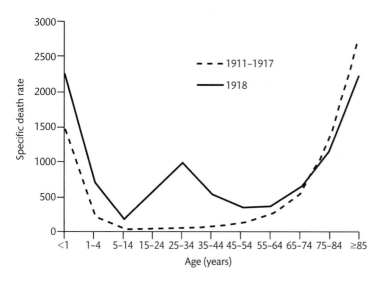

Figure 9.2 Age-specific mortality rates in the influenza epidemics of 1911–1917 and the so-called Spanish flu epidemic of 1918. The high virulence of the 1918 virus may have resulted from an aberrant host response; previous exposure of older persons to an antigenically related virus several decades earlier may explain the high mortality in younger people (from Taubenberger, J.K. and Morens, D.M. (2006) *Emerging Infectious Diseases* **12**, 15–22).

bacterium *Salmonella typhi*, which causes 21 million cases of typhoid and 200 000 deaths a year, principally in developing countries, although sporadic outbreaks do occur in developed countries, usually from contaminated food. What factors will influence its spread? People may vary in their sensitivity: this may place selective pressure on the population. Those with reduced immune function will be a particular risk: the elderly, young children, and those on immunosuppressant therapies or with immune deficiency diseases. Those previously exposed may have developed some immunity as will those immunized against the organism. But there will also be issues which relate to the bacterium itself. Clearly one aspect will be the strain involved in the outbreak, because selection has favoured the existence of different strains of *Salmonella* in the course of its contact with humans; genetic data shows that the ancestral strain of *S. typhi*, from which all other strains derive, still exists today. It probably arose after humans migrated from Africa and before the Neolithic period. But other strains have arisen since, and especially in the last 50 years, because they been exposed to the selection pressures of an environment laden with antibiotics and thus have developed resistance to the antibiotics which we have designed to treat ourselves. But different strains may have different virulence. Thus the survival and spread of the bacterium will depend on several things. A virulent strain will cause extreme symptoms in an affected person, and the resulting diarrhoea might produce a rapid spread of the bacterium. But the organism could also be a far less virulent strain, one which resides chronically in relatively symptomless carriers, not spread rapidly through high-intensity dispersal but slowly and continuously over a long period of time (see Box 9.6).

Box 9.6 Typhoid Mary

One of the most famous cases of a symptomless typhoid carrier is that of Mary Mallon, better known as Typhoid Mary. Originally from Ireland, she emigrated as a 15-year-old to the USA in 1884. In 1906, she was hired as a cook by a family during their summer vacation at a rented home. Shortly after, six of the 11 members in the house became hospitalized with typhoid fever. The alarmed landlords of the house sought the expertise of George Soper, a sanitation engineer, to determine the cause of the outbreak and salvage the reputation of their rental property. Soper discovered that Mallon's job history was strongly associated with incidences of typhoid fever. In fact a total of 22 people became infected at seven of her previous jobs, with one death recorded. Mallon herself was healthy and asymptomatic, and had no inkling that she could have been a carrier since such a concept was not known at the time. Her job as a cook increased her risk of infecting others.

Soper tracked Mallon down, requesting blood and stool samples so he could confirm the presence of the bacteria. Not surprisingly, Mallon was angry and appalled, and rebuffed several attempts to obtain samples until she was forcibly taken into custody. After stool analysis showed up typhoid bacteria, she was quarantined in an isolated cottage. In 1910, Mallon was freed on the condition that she did not work as a cook again. She performed domestic services but, never having been convinced of her status as a carrier, soon returned to cooking jobs under a pseudonym. However, 5 years later, Mallon was found to be responsible for an outbreak of typhoid fever in a Manhattan hospital. Her apparent recalcitrance won her no favours, and she was sent to quarantine again for the remainder of her life, a further 23 years. It is important to put Mallon's role in the spread of typhoid fever into perspective. There were about 50 other symptomless carriers known to the local health department at that time, and 3000 cases in New York state (including 600 fatalities) in 1906 alone. In contrast, just 33 cases and three fatalities have been attributed to Mallon. Some speculate that she has been immortalized in history books simply because of her stubbornness and the dramatic nature of her fight against health authorities.

Some diseases, particularly some that affect children such as measles, confer lifelong immunity in survivors. Because the measles virus has not apparently evolved a strain which can escape human immune responses, it is thought that it arose in the human form relatively recently, perhaps evolving within the last 20 000 years by transmission from cattle affected by a closely related morbillivirus, rinderpest. Measles was confined to Eurasia until the sixteenth century. Its conveyance to the Americas at that time produced devastating effects in the indigenous population which had no herd immunity, and it has been estimated that 95% of the indigenous Native American population was exterminated by such diseases. Why hasn't measles escaped from natural and acquired immunity to develop forms which reinfect us throughout our lives, just like influenza virus or the common cold?

9.3.4 Antibiotic resistance

The problem of antibiotic resistance is considerable although fears that a bacterial strain with multiple resistance to all known antibiotics could arise with disastrous consequences may be overstated: remember that the major improvements in death from infectious disease occurred in the pre-antibiotic era as a result of advances in vaccination, nutrition, and sanitation. The origins of antibiotic resistance are another consequence of human manipulation of the environment. Over-use through unnecessary prescribing is the major cause, but antibiotics are also used in animal feedstuffs and even impregnated into some children's toys.

How does antibiotic resistance evolve? Most antibiotics are derivatives of naturally occurring compounds that have evolved in micro-organisms as defences against other micro-organisms; the classic example is the production of penicillin by the mould *Penicillium*. The evolution of these defensive chemicals place selective pressure on the targeted micro-organism – and of course the producing organism must itself be resistant to its own antibiotic – and all microbial defence mechanisms, and their countermeasures, will have been tested by millions of years of selection. This implies that resistance mechanisms against most if not all naturally derived antibiotic classes will have evolved already, and indeed one of the major mechanisms by which bacteria acquire antibiotic resistance is the plasmid-mediated transfer from another

species of a resistance gene not previously found in the strain. Additionally, the large population size and short generation time of bacteria mean that new mutations conferring antibiotic resistance will occur frequently even within the human host. Such new mutations will be selected by contact with antibiotics.

Clinically relevant levels of resistance usually evolve within 2–4 years of the introduction of a new class of antibiotic (Figure 9.3). The mechanism underlying the resistance generally involves denying the antibiotic access to its target site. For example, this could be by the acquisition of degradative enzymes such as β-lactamases or of efflux pumps that remove the antibiotic from the bacterial cell, or reducing the sensitivity of the target site to the antibiotic, such as point mutations in the active sites of the DNA-replicating enzymes inhibited by the quinolone antibiotics such as ciprofloxacin.

Hospital-associated (nosocomial) infection with resistant bacteria is a particular threat. This is related to high rates of antibiotic use within the hospital setting, generating strong selective pressure favouring resistant strains and clearing sensitive strains, making colonization of patients and staff by resistant strains more likely. In addition, the high turnover of patients at the hospital imposes selective pressure for a resistant strain to transmit rapidly so as to remain endemic within the hospital.

Development and maintenance of antibiotic resistance will impose costs on the micro-organism; for example, associated with the production of degradative enzymes or the use of alternative, and less efficient, metabolic pathways to that targeted by the antibiotic. The hope that these costs would reduce the fitness of resistant strains sufficiently that they would be out-competed by more sensitive strains has not been fulfilled: compensatory mutations occur that restore fitness without loss of resistance. This implies that more rational use of antibiotics will not necessarily lead to a reduction in antibiotic resistance.

9.3.5 Microbiota and the human genome

All selective events are by definition reflected in the genome, but our long co-existence with viruses and bacteria shows special features. At the most fundamental level, mitochondria result from the successful invasion of a simple bacterium-like organism into a primitive

Antibiotic deployment

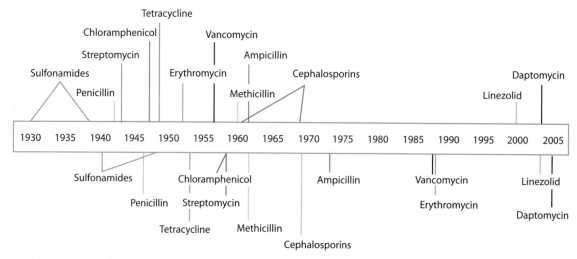

Antibiotic resistance observed

Figure 9.3 Timeline of antibiotic deployment and the development of antibiotic resistance. Note the rapid appearance of resistance after deployment (from Clatworthy, A.E. *et al.* (2007) *Nature Chemical Biology* **3**, 541–548, with permission).

eukaryote, probably 2–3 billion years ago at around the time free oxygen first became available in the atmosphere. An intracellular cohabitation – endosymbiosis – evolved by which cellular functions became divided between nuclear genetic control and that of the bacterium, which became limited to respiratory functions. Most of the genes of the bacterium have been transferred to the host's nuclear genome, and the remaining 16 568 base pairs (in the human reference sequence) encode the 37 remaining genes of the mitochondrial genome.

Retroviruses are RNA-based viruses with an enzyme, reverse transcriptase, which copies the viral RNA to its complementary DNA and this allows the virus to be replicated by the host DNA. Retroviruses have evolved two distinct strategies: that of exogenous infection as in the case of lentiviruses such as HIV, and that of invasion of the germ cell line. These endogenous retroviruses thus become part of the genomic DNA and are passed through the germ line to future generations. It is estimated that 8% of human genomic DNA consists of such endogenous retroviruses but if we extend this to fragments and altered sequences of ancient retroviruses, it might amount to as much as half of our DNA. Almost all of these viral inserts

are now harmless, although some retrotransposon-induced mutations can produce evolutionarily or clinically relevant effects on gene expression (see Chapter 3).

The selective effects of infectious agents on humans may cause harmful alleles to be retained within the population because of balancing selection (see Chapter 3), where an allele may be harmful in the homozygous state but have some advantage in the heterozygous state; thus an equilibrium is reached between the normal and mutant alleles.

9.3.6 Innate immunity

All multicellular animals possess an innate immune system, which protects from infection by maintaining defensive barriers against penetration by micro-organisms and by mounting non-specific chemical and cellular defences against microbes that do reach the interior of the organism. Innate immunity is non-specific and, unlike the adaptive immune system (see below) does not lead to any lasting protective immunity (or 'memory'). The innate immune system is phylogenetically ancient, and many of its features are conserved across both vertebrates and invertebrates.

The physical barriers that resist invasion by micro-organisms include the skin as well as the mucous membranes lining the alimentary tract and parts of the respiratory and reproductive tracts. These barriers are equipped with sensory receptors which are deployed at strategic points, where they have greater sensitivity. On the most often exposed parts of our skin such as the fingers and face, sensitivity is greatest; mechanoreceptors can detect very small inhaled particles in the nose or larynx. Tight junctions at the cells provide good protection against the passage of micro-organisms; the waterproofing of the skin limits passage of water-borne organisms and the mucus-secreting glands and ciliary action of the mucous membranes helps to expel ingested or inhaled organisms. Some attackers have evolved with highly effective ways of penetrating these barriers, such as the proboscis of the mosquito, and other parasites such as the malaria protozoan use this as a way of gaining access.

Other barriers within the body have different degrees of penetrability and defensive strategies. The human placenta, for example, is somewhat 'leaky', prioritizing exchange and transport functions over defence, and so some micro-organisms such as the syphilis spirochaete (*Treponema pallidum*), rubella virus, *Toxoplasma gondii*, *Listeria bacteroides*, and cytomegalovirus can pass from mother to fetus. At the other extreme the barrier between blood and brain is very tight except for the cribriform plate (which conducts the olfactory nerves from the nose) and this provides a route for infection leading to meningitis. Amoebic meningitis, a very rare disease, can arise when contaminated water found in natural hot springs enters the nose.

The next line of defence is provided by inflammatory and phagocytic cells, such as macrophages and neutrophils, and by the antimicrobial substances they secrete, such as complement. The triggering of these defences to invading organisms involves recognition of chemical structures, called pathogen-associated molecular patterns (PAMPs), that are common to micro-organisms but not found on more complex animals. In other words, this form of discrimination between self and non-self takes the form of a generalized ability to distinguish between multicellular and single-celled organisms. PAMPs include bacterial cell wall molecules such as lipopolysaccharides as well as unmethylated DNA (as described in Chapter 4, most eukaryotic DNA is methylated).

Competition for the essential nutrient iron illustrates the interaction between host and invader. Microbial growth in host tissues is limited by the availability of free iron, and infection induces secretion by the host of iron-binding proteins such as transferrin, which act to sequester iron intracellularly and make it unavailable for bacterial metabolism. For their part, bacteria secrete siderophores, which are small peptides that bind iron and transport it into their cells. In turn, the host processes that detect PAMPs stimulate the secretion of a small protein called lipocalin 2, which binds the bacterial siderophores with very high affinity and deprives the pathogens of iron. In experimental animals the absence of this defence mechanism can result in sepsis and death. Infection-associated anaemia is a common clinical finding, particularly with chronic infection, leading to the question of whether iron supplementation in such situations is deleterious or beneficial.

Bacteria have evolved ways of fighting back against every defence which hosts have devised. This includes secreting toxins which inhibit ciliary action or the production of a protective biofilm. The invasion of the body can involve the use of syringe-like mechanisms to gain entry to cells, thus avoiding surface defences. Many bacteria shield themselves from the PAMP recognition system by secreting masking molecules which block antigen recognition (see below) on infected cells and alter pro-inflammatory cytokine or antibody production.

There are many other forms of defence which micro-organisms can use to overcome the responses of the host. One example is the contingency loci found in several genera of bacterial pathogens. These loci, usually associated with genes that interact in some way with the host, such as a membrane protein, contain short sequence repeats analogous to the microsatellites found in eukaryotes (Chapter 3). These repeats are randomly and reversibly hypermutable, causing genotypic switching at these loci and therefore high phenotypic diversity that enables the pathogen to evade host responses. A somewhat similar process is used by the trypanosomes that cause sleeping sickness to generate the variant surface glycoproteins (VSGs) that act as decoys for the host immune response, although here the variants arise from an archive of pre-existing *VSG* genes rather than from *de novo* mutations. A final example is provided by the extreme diversity in the envelope proteins and drug-target molecules of HIV, which is caused by the low fidelity of the virus's reverse transcriptase.

9.3.7 Adaptive immunity

Beyond the innate immune system, the adaptive immune system is the key weapon in the vertebrate war against microbial infection. The adaptive immune system differs from the innate immune system in two general ways. First, it is able to respond to any macromolecule that is perceived by the individual as non-self rather than to a non-specific pattern signalling the presence of a pathogen. Second, although the initial response of the adaptive immune system to a new challenge is relatively weak, it has a 'memory' that ensures that subsequent encounters with the same molecule cause faster and stronger responses than the first challenge. It is this second feature that causes the adaptive immune system to be so named. The adaptive immune system provides vertebrates with a powerful defence against microbial infection, and with immune surveillance against aberrant clones of its own cells, but its exquisite specificity has two clinically relevant consequences: susceptibility to autoimmune and atopic disease, and rejection of transplanted tissue.

The ability to discriminate between self and non-self is critical to the function of the adaptive immune system, and defects in this process of **immunological tolerance** underlie autoimmune disease. The fundamental basis of recognition of self or non-self macromolecules by the adaptive immune system is the display of fragments of those molecules on the cell surface bound to proteins of the **major histocompatibility complex** (MHC). There are two classes of MHC molecule: nearly all cells express class I, which displays fragments of the normal proteins of the cell, allowing the immune system to detect whether the cell's protein synthetic machinery has been subverted by viral infection or tumourigenesis. Conversely, class II molecules are expressed only by specialized antigen-presenting cells, which phagocytose and degrade micro-organisms and display protein fragments from foreign antigens. Recognition of a displayed peptide as non-self by a T cell triggers an immune response: in general, recognition of non-self in the context of MHC class I causes a cell-mediated response that kills the subverted cell, whereas recognition in the context of MHC class II causes both a cell-mediated and an antibody-mediated response.

The multi-subunit MHC molecules are coded for by genes on chromosome 6, each of which have extraordinarily wide (up to several hundred alleles) diversity, much of which is expressed at the peptide-binding site of the molecule. This combination of allelic variation and subunit pairing means that the resulting MHC complexes are capable of binding a huge variety of different peptides. Such genetic diversity is best explained by balancing selection driven by the different ability of particular MHC alleles to protect against particular pathogens. Even in a small population, there will be many different MHC allele combinations that protect against the multiple pathogens in the environment and thwart the evolution of new pathogen epitopes.

Box 9.7   The MHC: more than just immunology

While the MHC comprises an integral part of the body's immune defence system, it also serves another function which, superficially, appears unrelated: it contributes to an individual's 'signature' scent, or body odour. Studies on animals ranging from fish to humans have revealed that the scents emitted differ from individual to individual and are highly dependent on MHC genotype. In mice, scents originate from specific combinations of volatile metabolites present in urine, and the detection of olfactory differences enables mice to recognize each other. Less is known about the nature of body scents emitted by humans, but it seems that the ability to discriminate between scents plays a role in sexual attraction, and therefore mate selection.

How does this link with the immunological function of MHC? A Swiss group performed an intriguing experiment in which men were asked to wear t-shirts for two consecutive nights and forego scented toiletries. The sweat-stained t-shirts were collected, and women were then asked to rate the 'pleasantness' of the odours. The researchers found that the women tended to prefer odours from men who were MHC-dissimilar to themselves. These results could be explained by mate preference being driven by the need to ensure that offspring have increased MHC heterozygosity, as this may be vital in disease resistance. Also, selecting a genetically dissimilar mate could be a means of reducing the chances of inbreeding.

These notions are supported by studies on the Hutterite religious clan, a closed self-sufficient group whose members only marry within-clan. Even though the gene pool is more limited in this community, couplings nevertheless tended to be between MHC-dissimilar members, and the couples that did share MHC similarity were more likely to have higher rates of miscarriage and difficulty conceiving.

The exact evolutionary reasons for the involvement of MHC genotype in mating preferences in humans and other animals still remain somewhat speculative. Nevertheless the association is consistently strong and elucidation of the basis by which the MHC modulates odour production could provide further clues on the nature of human chemical communication.

In humans, the MHC system is also known as the **human leucocyte antigen** (HLA) system. The HLA system is the predominant determinant of tissue compatibility after transplantation and the wide diversity of HLA alleles makes tissue rejection likely unless careful matching is performed. Another situation where tolerance between HLA-incompatible individuals is critical is at the materno–fetal interface. The fetal trophoblast cells that contact maternal tissues during pregnancy do not express classical MHC class I or II molecules on their surface, and instead express a set of minor HLA genes with restricted allele diversity and immunosuppressive properties towards maternal cells.

Two facets of the adaptive immune system represent selection at a suborganismic level. First, recognition of self antigens is central for immunological tolerance and the avoidance of autoimmune disease. The 'education' of the immune system to distinguish self from non-self is a selective process that takes place in the thymus during development. Immature T cells, each of which carries a T cell receptor on its surface that binds to just one of the estimated 10 million different types of epitope recognized by the human immune system, are normally programmed to undergo apoptosis and die shortly after they are formed. In the thymus, they are exposed to the full range of self antigens, and those that fail to react are 'rescued' from the apoptotic process and released into the blood. This 'fail-safe' mechanism ensures that the organism develops with a set of T cells that respond only to foreign antigens.

The second process is the clonal expansion of B cells. During their development, each B cell is programmed to produce a single one of the wide range of possible immunoglobulins, and this is displayed on its surface as part of the B cell receptor. Once released into the circulation, if it encounters that epitope it is stimulated to proliferate, leading to the production of millions of identical B cells that secrete immunoglobulins with the correct specificity. In the course of this clonal expansion, further fine-tuning of immunoglobulin specificity occurs by a process of somatic hypermutation, which promotes erroneous DNA repair and increases the mutation rate in the variable region of the immunoglobulin gene by about a million-fold. The resulting variations in immunoglobulin amino acid sequence are random, but only those cells with the highest affinity for antigen are selected to survive and proliferate. The end results of this Darwinian-like process of variation and selection, termed affinity maturation, are two-fold: plasma cells that secrete large amounts of immunoglobulin of high specificity and the development of memory B cells containing the relevant DNA sequence that persist for years in lymph nodes and are activated rapidly on new exposure to the antigen.

Box 9.8   Transgenerational passage of acquired immune characteristics

After birth the human neonate must defend itself against micro-organisms, but there is a daunting array of them. The lactating mother can help. Of the five classes of human antibody, IgA dominates in breast milk. IgA antibodies are able to confer a considerable degree of passive immunity on the baby, in a system with a high degree of efficiency. The antibodies are produced only by the mother, in response to organisms which she encounters, and which are likely to be highly relevant to her baby too, but they do not harm the developing bacterial flora of the infant's gut which are needed for digestion. The first milk, colostrum, produced by the mother also contains interferon, which inhibits viral growth. This is non-specific as all viruses are unhelpful at this age. Another helpful series of compounds in the milk are oligosaccharides, simple sugars which contain copies of the binding sites by which bacteria gain entry into the body's cells. Thus they are helpful in binding to bacteria in the gut and making them more likely to be destroyed by antibodies and macrophages. Other factors in milk include lactoferrin which interferes with bacterial iron metabolism, bifidus factor which promotes the growth of the beneficial commensal *Lactobacillus bifidus*, and fibronectin which makes macrophages more aggressive. In addition, breast milk contains both macrophages and antibody-producing leucocytes, again their activities tuned by the exposure of the mother. They can remain active in the infant's gut for several weeks, allowing time for the infant's immune responses to mature.

9.3.8 Vaccination

Vaccination, together with improved nutrition and sanitation, underlies the decrease in morbidity from infectious disease that has occurred in high-income countries over the last 100 years. Two issues merit consideration in the context of an evolutionary perspective: first, whether existing vaccines are likely to become ineffective in the face of evolutionary change, and second whether an understanding of bacterial and viral evolution can assist in the design of new vaccines.

Vaccination has eradicated one human disease (smallpox), is close to eradicating another (poliomyelitis), and in the developed world controls several acute childhood infections, such as rubella and measles (Figure 9.4). These diseases are the 'easy' ones in that natural infection with these agents, if not fatal, generally provides lifelong immunity against a second infection. Viral evolution has failed to break through the lifelong natural immunity conferred by the initial infection, and there is no evidence to suggest that the situation would be different in relation to vaccine-induced immunity against these pathogens.

However, there are several examples of existing human and veterinary vaccines where evolution of the targeted organism has been demonstrated in response to the selection pressure of the vaccine, and in the case of one veterinary product (against Marek's disease, a virus-induced neoplasia in poultry) this has led to large-scale failure of the vaccine. How might an organism respond to a vaccine? First, it might evolve by selection against the epitopes recognized by vaccine-induced immunity. Such epitope shifting, potentially leading to loss of vaccine effectiveness, has been observed for several human viral and bacterial vaccines including those for hepatitis B, pertussis, and pneumococcal disease. Second, it might evolve with a change in virulence. Recall from the discussion of virulence above that a pathogen will evolve to a level of virulence that optimizes its transmission, balancing the cost of early death of the host against the benefit of high virulence and therefore high transmission. If vaccination acts to reduce the death rate of the host, then selection might act on the pathogen to favour an increase in its virulence, because this will increase the chance of transmission and thus the fitness of the pathogen. Consequently, the disease will become more severe in unvaccinated hosts. At a population level, pathogen evolution of this kind may negate the benefit of a vaccination

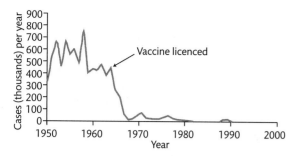

Figure 9.4 Reported cases of measles in the USA, 1950–2001. Note the rapid drop in disease incidence after the licensing of the vaccine in 1963 (from Centers for Disease Control, www.cdc.gov/vaccines/vac-gen/6mishome.htm).

programme by increasing the cost of managing the disease in unprotected individuals. The failure of the Marek's disease vaccine in chickens was caused by vaccine-driven increases in viral virulence.

Current vaccine development is aimed at the 'difficult' diseases where selection has already partially overcome host immunity against the pathogen so that repeat infection is possible (for example, influenza) or indeed where host immunity inevitably fails and initial infection becomes chronic (such as HIV or malaria). In the case of influenza, epitope shifting in wild-type organisms requires continuous surveillance of strains and regular reformulation of the vaccine. In the second case, within-host epitope shifting requires that vaccines be targeted at invariant, functionally essential epitopes and/or at multiple epitopes. The difficulty of this enterprise is illustrated by the failure, in spite of decades of effort, to develop vaccines against these diseases.

9.3.9 Dysregulation of the immune system

9.3.9.1 Autoimmune disease
Diseases in which the immune system attacks the body's own cells, as if mistaking them for non-self pathogens, are termed autoimmune diseases. There are genomic characteristics that can affect the potential to develop autoimmune disease, usually associated with particular alleles of the HLA system. For example, HLA-DR2 is associated with systemic lupus erythematosus, which is more common in females, and ankylosing spondylitis is associated with HLA-B27 and is more common among males.

Ankylosing spondylitis develops gradually during adolescence and young adulthood, causing chronic inflammation and structural changes in joints, especially in the spine. But not all HLA-B27 males develop the disease, so there must be some other environmental trigger. There is some evidence to suggest that the trigger in some cases is a response to *Klebsiella* commensals which inhabit the gut, perhaps itself triggered by an acute infection, since there are cross-reacting epitopes between *Klebsiella* and human cell-surface antigens.

9.3.9.2 Developmental regulation of immunity
The interaction between nutrition and infection is particularly important in developing countries, and especially in children. An early effect of malnutrition is suppression of immune function. For example, in a population of subsistence farmers in The Gambia with highly seasonal food availability, people born in the 'hungry season' showed 10-fold higher infection-related mortality as young adults, suggesting that immune function may be compromised by events early in life. In this population, thymus development was sensitive to early-life nutrition, with smaller thymuses observed in those born in the hungry season. Furthermore, size at birth was positively correlated with antibody responses to vaccination. Such observations may represent the results of trade-offs in which the body prioritizes resource use and favours immediate survival over investment in long-term defence mechanisms (see Chapter 5).

9.3.9.3 Allergies and chronic inflammatory disorders
We have seen repeatedly in this book that environmental change which produces evolutionary novelty can pose a threat to human health. In contrast to the fall in morbidity from infectious diseases seen in developed countries over the past 100 years or so, the prevalence of asthma, allergies, and chronic inflammatory disorders such as Crohn's disease has increased dramatically (Figure 9.5). One explanation relates to the changes in the type of pathogens that humans are exposed to. For example, there is a lower prevalence of asthma and atopic disorders in children in rural compared with urban communities. Inflammatory bowel disease is common in highly sanitized, industrialized areas of the world, but uncommon in rural areas where living quarters are crowded and unhygienic. Breastfeeding in infants has a protective effect

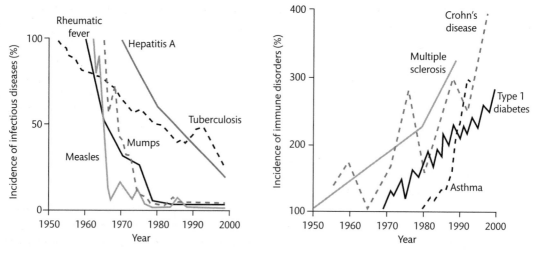

Figure 9.5 As the incidence of infectious disease has fallen in high-income countries, the incidence of immune-related disorders has increased (from Bach, J.-F. (2002) *New England Journal of Medicine* **347**, 911–920, with permission).

in reducing the later risk of asthma, possibly because of the different types of bacterial flora to which breast- and bottle-fed infants are exposed. Germ-free mice experience abnormal development of their immune system, which can be corrected by re-introduction of intestinal commensal bacteria or even by administration of purified polysaccharides from those bacteria.

A proposed unifying mechanism, termed the **hygiene hypothesis**, is that the vertebrate adaptive immune system has co-evolved with both commensal and pathogenic micro-organisms, and that appropriate exposure to this microbiota early in life is essential to set up immunoregulatory pathways. Lack of such exposure leads to inappropriate activation of immune responses which are then manifest as allergic or autoimmune responses.

One candidate for such an immunoregulatory-inducing organism is helminthic worms. Intestinal infestation with helminthic worms was nearly universal in human evolutionary history, but is now rare in high-income countries. Although infestation with helminths can cause IgE-mediated responses, the organisms are difficult to clear and the host tends to develop tolerance rather than mounting a futile and self-damaging immune reaction. Experimental studies show that helminthic infestation is protective against a number of immune-mediated diseases. Clinical trials involving deliberate helminth infestation of patients with inflammatory bowel disease (the pig

whipworm, *Trichuris suis*, was used since it is not pathogenic in humans) reduced disease activity in patients with ulcerative colitis and Crohn's disease.

An alternative view is that new environments provide specific risk factors that were absent from older environments. For example, our homes are now much drier and warmer than they used to be, often with fitted carpets, warm bedding, and central heating. This provides an ideal environment for mites which inhabit house dust, their food source being sloughed human skin. The faeces of these mites are highly allergenic in susceptible people.

9.4 Other threats

Other organisms also injure humans, such as poisonous snakes, spiders, scorpions, and jellyfish. The potentially lethal effects of these organisms occur because they are defending themselves against perceived attack by us, using mechanisms which they evolved with to kill or immobilize their own prey. These species have evolved the capacity to make and secrete highly effective toxins which target fundamental physiological mechanisms, usually neural communication, to deadly effect. While evolving such poisons is a highly effective strategy for these predators in obtaining their food and defending themselves, we have not evolved defences against them

CHAPTER 10

Social organization and behaviour

10.1 Introduction

It is a truism that humans can be distinguished, at least in degree, from other species by a large brain relative to body size. Our brain is characterized by a particularly well-developed neocortex and this has had a number of profound evolutionary consequences. Our capacity to communicate, to use and develop technology, and even the nature of the social structures we have evolved, can be attributed to a large neocortex. Humans are a social species. We evolved with characteristic behaviours adapted to live in groups with others of our species. Yet our societal structure has undergone enormous change in a few thousand years, from the small isolated clan of many foraging societies to the complex organizations of cities with populations in the millions. Increasingly, the social environment is changing in other ways. Family structure has changed, and communication is no longer necessarily verbal and face to face; indeed, telephone, radio, television, and the internet are now all dominant forms of communication.

This chapter considers how human behaviour has evolved and how this has impacted on behavioural morbidity as reflected in psychological and psychiatric disorders. These forms of disorders are now an enormous component of the current and anticipated burden of disease. The social environment is a major component of the selective environment which has led to the evolution of our species. But at the same time, humans have evolved with a rapidly changing capacity to alter their social and societal environments. This creates the potential for a mismatch between our evolved phenotype and the environment we now inhabit. This, in turn, is a potent source of psychological disorder.

10.2 Biological determinants of culture and behaviour

Culture is generally defined as an amalgam of knowledge, behaviour, and tradition within a particular community or population. But creating a formal definition of 'culture' has itself been contentious. There have been intense debates among the social science disciplines over its precise definition. Some have argued that culture must be viewed as a purely human characteristic, but there are cultural phenomena observed in other species. For example, there can be quite distinct patterns of tool use in different chimpanzee clans and there is evidence of cultural transmission of behaviours in a variety of primates.

It is obvious that human culture evolves, and this **cultural evolution** is another form of an inheritance system with the potential for both vertical and horizontal transmission (see Chapter 2). Understanding the significance of the interplay between organic and cultural evolution is important. The evolution of the capacity to learn and the potential for learning to influence evolution are also important components of evolutionary science. But what has to be learned – and how it is learned – has changed dramatically and rapidly in the past 5000 years, from experiential learning within the forager clan to formalized and structured learning.

Because of varying attitudes to what culture is and how it originates, evolutionary explanations of human behaviour have had an especially contentious history. This contention arose in part because of philosophical and political debate stemming from how various disciplines have interpreted human behaviour. Some have wanted to view it as an entirely learned phenomenon, while other disciplines argue, in our view self-evidently, that human behaviour is built on some strongly selected and therefore genetically determined components of brain function. Extreme positions have been taken, or at least been interpreted as being taken, and at times the debate has been polemic and uncritical. The media has not infrequently exaggerated scientific reasoning and observations into fatuous extrapolations.

We can reduce this discourse to the fundamental question of to what extent human behaviour is determined (or influenced) by our evolved biology. Several schools of conceptual thought (see Box 10.4, below) emerged to explain the evolution of human behaviour, largely based on how each conceived of culture, behaviour, and learning. The debate was distorted by the strong genetic determinism of late-twentieth-century biology. The distinguished evolutionary biologist and zoologist E.O. Wilson, and subsequently many others including Richard Dawkins, put forward deterministic arguments in which all aspects of behaviour were essentially framed in genetic (i.e. evolved) terms. Their critics, perhaps unfairly, saw that this stance left little room for the role of active decision-making, learning, and cultural adaptation. At its most inappropriate extreme, these critics saw biological arguments being used to excuse all forms of anti-social behaviours from rape to murder, a position exploited by the media and a gross misuse of the evolutionary arguments.

Social sciences take a very different view to the biological perspective: they see human behaviour as being dominated by culture that is learned from others. The basis of social science is that humans are cultural organisms, and in general social scientists perceive culture as a learned rather than innate phenomenon. They argue that humans are quantitatively *and* qualitatively different from other species in terms of the complexity of our culture.

But culture itself is a product of evolution, and culture is not a uniquely human characteristic. Learning can be demonstrated in many animals. For example, some

aspects of foraging are clearly learned, feeding behaviours are culturally transmitted in some reptiles and birds, migratory patterns are learned in some avian species, and tool use in different groups of chimpanzees is a learned or culturally transmitted behaviour. Language provides a sophisticated capacity for communication and we have developed varied and complex social structures. We are a prescient species with a consciousness, we use technology in sophisticated ways and we have developed belief systems manifesting in religion and superstition. But there is an important difference between the views that genes determine our behaviour and the argument that our evolved brain is the substrate on which experience and the current environment shape our abilities and behaviour.

A fair appraisal of the concepts would show that accepting that there is a genetic basis to human behaviour does not mean that every aspect of human behaviour is genetically determined (evolved). Rather, as we have made clear throughout this book, genetic factors provide a substrate on which developmental and environmental influences (including the social components of the environment) act to mould behavioural and neural phenotypes. It is this summation which would be a fair assessment of where the field of evolutionary analysis of behaviour is now positioned.

Evolutionary arguments satisfactorily explain both how altruistic behaviour and the interplay between the sexes has emerged. In this chapter we will extend the discussion to other aspects of human behaviour and psychology. But each of these schools of thought offers valuable insights, and this chapter will draw from them to describe what is now a broadly held consensus on how evolutionary principles can, and should, be used to explain human behaviour and psychology. In turn, evolutionary perspectives do offer some useful insights into understanding psychiatric disorders.

10.3 Evolution of human brain and behaviour

In considering the evolution of human behaviour it is useful to bear in mind the four questions suggested by Tinbergen as way of systematically understanding behaviour and which were reviewed in Chapter 1. These were: what is the mechanism underpinning the behaviour, what is the function of the behaviour, how does it develop during the life course, and how does it evolve? Addressing each of these questions are components of fully understanding behaviour from both a proximate and ultimate perspective.

Primates have brain sizes relative to body size about an order of magnitude larger than that of other mammals. But even within the primate order, humans and our ancestor species have had brain sizes that are disproportionately large (see Chapter 6). The investment in a large brain size has major energetic considerations. The human brain consumes about 20% of total energy consumption while constituting about 2% of bodyweight and the proportion is considerably higher in the infant. So a fundamental evolutionary question is why primates, and particularly hominins, evolved investing so much of their energetic resources into brain growth and function. The question does not have a single unitary answer.

The simple answer is that the sensory and processing capacities of the brain conferred adaptive advantages to the primate clade. For example, primates use senses such as colour vision to a greater extent than other mammals in their search for ripe fruits. Evolutionary processes do not work on a single trait in isolation, but operate on multiple interacting traits. Indeed there has been an interactive 'ratchet' involving changing ecology, evolving social structure, better communication, and better use of technology, all of which have driven brain development.

One thesis put forward by Robin Dunbar is that primates found advantage in living in groups with a complex social structure. This enabled them to defend against predators and to defend food supply in larger territories. But living in a large group requires a complex dynamic among the individuals because of the social complexity that ensues. Neocortical volumes correlate strongly with group size in primates (see Chapter 6); in humans the neocortical volume is approximately 80% of total brain size, whereas it is much less in some prosimians. Based on these relationships, Dunbar proposed that humans evolved living in group sizes of about 150 individuals. Intriguingly, modern forager societies tend to be built around clans of this group size. Early villages and those

in modern agricultural societies (and even communes) tend to be of similar size. Sociological research shows that group sizes of about 150 are the maximum before complex hierarchies are required. Sociological research suggests that while people in modern societies may have many more 'acquaintances', perhaps up to 2000 individuals, the circle of true friends, intimate acquaintances, and relatives averages about 150 people (see Table 6.1). Language appears to be the tool that allows humans to manage the complex interactions of group sizes of this nature. In contrast, chimpanzees and other primates live in group sizes of 50 or less, and other forms of interaction such as grooming may play an important role in ensuring social cohesion in these groups. Likewise, cuddling remains an important element in maintaining relationships in human families.

Social complexity within a group requires the capacity of each member to interpret the **intentionality** of others within the group. This is not simply a matter of communication. It is a matter of interpreting intent and understanding not only the relationship between two individuals, but all the potential relationships within a group. An analytical construct has been developed to describe how animals and humans interpret the mental state and intentionality of others within the species: this is termed the **theory of mind**. This construct provides an analytical basis for how communication and social interaction can move beyond simple alarm calls and herd behaviour to the complexities of human society and culture. It explains how one individual assesses the thoughts of another and responds to them.

But such advanced processing and engagement in social organization clearly required, and was expedited by, the development of language (see Chapter 6). Once higher levels of intentionality had evolved, they provided the capacity for further components of human culture to develop. They also provided the basis for a high level of reciprocal altruism and cheater detection, which have become fundamental to the structure of human society. Higher levels of intentionality are required for the capacity to have prescient self awareness (including that of death), to develop belief and superstition (the forerunners of ritual and religion), to form political structures and to use language to communicate via the complexities and beauty of poetry.

Box 10.1 Theory of mind

This evolutionary psychological construct is used to describe how members of a species interact when interpreting each others' behaviour and thoughts. It is directly linked to neocortical capacity and function. It is also useful in understanding how the human's ability to interact develops from infancy to adulthood. There is a close relationship between these concepts and that of consciousness: the ability to assess one's own state of mind and that of others.

The basis of theory of mind is a hierarchy of *orders of intentionality*.

1 I am aware of my own thoughts: this is first-order intentionality.
2 I also think I can assess what a second person is thinking in an interaction: this is second-order intentionality.
3 But I might want to assess what that second person is thinking about me (in other words, what his second-order assessment of me is): this is third-order intentionality.
4 But then I might want to assess what that second person is thinking about how I think about what he is thinking: this is fourth-order intentionality.

This can continue, serving as the structure of adult human interactions. The more political our intent, the higher the levels of intentionality that we need to employ.

Many experiments have been performed to assess the level of intentionality in non-human primates. Some primates, mainly Old World socially advanced species such as baboons and macaques, clearly practise deception, particularly in relation to sexual matters, and sometimes food access. This requires third-order intentionality.

It is generally accepted that most adult humans operate with about five or six levels of intentionality. Indeed, effective social discourse requires this level of interaction to avoid unnecessary misunderstandings and conflict. Clearly the higher the level of intentionality required, the more likely errors of interaction will result. Many problems in interpersonal relationships and even wars have arisen as we employ these higher levels of intentionality. The theory of mind develops over our life course. By the age of 4–5, children can recognize a third-order of intentionality: before that they cannot lie convincingly. The concept of a theory of the mind may be relevant to understanding autism and the related Asperger's syndrome. Those afflicted have a limited ability to interpret the intent of others, suggesting that third-order and higher levels of intentionality have not developed appropriately.

10.4 Evolution of social behaviour

Humans are social animals. We are characterized by living in groups larger than our family and, as discussed previously, there is a rationale for the view that we evolved living in clans of about 150 individuals. Thus the social environment became a key part of our selective environment, and selection would have favoured traits which promoted fitness within the social environments that we evolved and lived within.

However, we also evolved in parallel with our cultural repertoire. There has been a close reciprocity between our cultural evolution and our biological evolution, often referred to as **gene–culture co-evolution**.

The development of tools by *Homo habilis* is the first unequivocal evidence of culture in the hominin clade. That tool-making capacity evolved through learning and cultural evolution into the technological repertoire of modern society such as brain scanning, pharmaceutical development, nuclear weapons, and the internet.

There are many features of society which have undergone change, many of which are self evident. Over the past 10 000 years, humans have changed from foragers living in small clans into pastoralists and city dwellers. These changes have been accompanied by rising exposures to infection and malnutrition (see Chapters 7 and 9). The causes and nature of trauma and conflict have also changed, with humans becoming our own main predators. There have also been enormous changes in social structure. Organizational and thus power hierarchies became necessary, and individual skills became differentiated: a surgeon and a lawyer have very different skills (at least they should have), and interpersonal interactions often now require higher levels of intentionality.

Culture evolves and as it changes so does the selective environment in which an individual lives. The example in Chapter 1 of how lactase persistence co-evolved with pastoralism demonstrates such co-evolution. Conversely, had the gene for lactase persistence not mutated, milk could not have become a major food source for that population. It is not surprising that the outcome of this duality may be maladaptive, because culture can evolve at a different pace and in a different manner to biological evolution. For example, the evolution of societal structure into large population aggregations with less structured clan support may be in conflict with our evolved capacity to manage best in smaller groups. This mismatch may be the basis of some psychological disorders. In Chapter 7 we described how the low age of biological puberty is in conflict with the age at which we accept young people as adults in developed societies. Indeed, it may be that the change in societal complexity has affected the rate of neural maturation: there being evidence that decision-making activity may not mature until about 20 years of age (Figure 10.1) and prefrontal cortical structures which are involved in impulse control, strategizing, and judgement are not fully mature until after 25 years of age (Figure 10.2). There is growing empirical evidence to show that this mismatch plays a role in teen-

age depression, acting-out behaviour, drug abuse, and suicide. Boys who underwent earlier puberty, spending a longer period of their lives in a biologically mature but psychologically immature phase, were much more likely to be suicidal than those who had biological puberty at later age (Table 10.1). This example highlights a challenge. Just as the introduction of an exotic species into a previously stable environment (for example, rats and humans in New Zealand, which was free of terrestrial mammals until the arrival of humans some 700 years ago) can drive species (the flightless moa) extinct, or as global warming can destroy frog habitats in the mountains of Costa Rica, rapid changes in our social environment can have impacts on human health. The human neocortex largely evolved to deal with the challenges of the social environment. As biological and cultural evolution proceed in very different ways and paces, we can anticipate that the consequences of the inevitable mismatch between brain and environment will be reflected in disorders of behaviour and mental health.

10.4.1 Altruism

One of the biggest challenges in evolutionary biology has been to explain altruism. Initially altruism was used as an argument for group selection, but problems were inherent in that concept (as discussed in Chapter 2) and it was abandoned. So if the unit of selection is the individual or the gene, how can behaviour that apparently does not serve the reproductive interests of the individual (i.e. altruism) evolve?

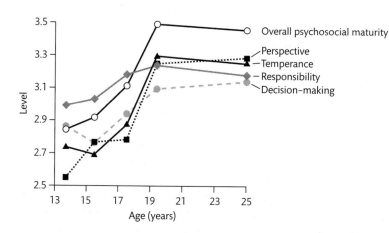

Figure 10.1 Decision-making activity may not mature until about 20 years of age (data from Cauffman, E. and Steinberg, L. (2000) *Behavioral Sciences and the Law* **18**, 741–760).

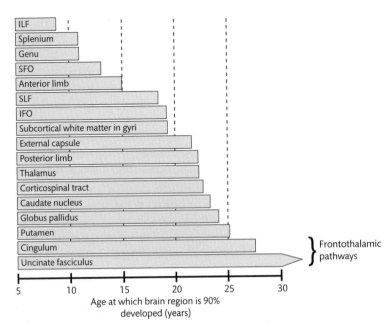

Figure 10.2 Magnetic resonance imaging of the human brain shows that frontothalamic structures, which are involved in impulse control, strategizing, and judgement, are not fully mature until late in the third decade of life. ILF, inferior longitudinal fasciculus; SFO, superior fronto-occipital fasciculus; SLF, superior longitudinal fasciculus; IFO, inferior fronto-occipital fasciculus (modified from Lebel, C. *et al.* (2008) *Neuroimage* **40**, 1044–1055, with permission).

Table 10.1 Early puberty increases the risk of psychological disturbance during adolescence. Odds ratios represent the increased risk conferred by early maturation compared with average timing of maturation

Area of risk	Odds ratio
Females	
Body-image concerns	1.3
Smoking	1.4
Functional symptoms	1.5
Victimization	1.7
Sexually active	1.9
Males	
Drunkenness in previous 6 months	1.4
Victimization	1.7
Cannabis usage	1.8
Sexually active	1.8
Smoking	1.8
Illegal drug usage	2.0
Depression	2.1
Functional symptoms	2.2
Suicide attempt	4.9

Data from Michaud, P.-A. *et al.* (2006) *Molecular and Cellular Endocrinology* **254–255**, 172–178.

Altruism is a common feature of mammalian systems. A meerkat will take up a guard position to watch for a predatory raptor even though this entails a greater risk of being spotted and becoming a victim. One member, not necessarily a parent, will guard the nest while others in the clan are out hunting. Much in human social behaviour appears to be for the benefit of others rather than for one's own selfish reproductive effort. As discussed in Chapter 2, a favoured explanation is provided in part by the concepts of kin selection and inclusive fitness.

William Hamilton, the originator of the concept of kin selection, argued that an animal would behave altruistically with respect to other animals if those other animals are likely to carry the same genes. That is, it is the intergenerational flow of genetic material that drives evolution. This would apply in the case of kin, and the closer the kinship, the more likely it is that altruistic behaviour would be beneficial. This is formulated in **Hamilton's rule**, which states that a gene supporting altruistic behaviour would be under positive selection whenever the benefit to the recipient of the altruistic act (in terms of offspring) is greater than the cost to the individual conducting the beneficial act. This is clearly dependent on the degree of relatedness: the greater the degree, the greater the benefit in terms of potential gene flow.

Indeed there is considerable empirical evidence that altrustic acts in animals are more likely when there is a high degree of relatedness. This concept of kin selection has also be used to explain the development of eusociality in insect species such as the honey bee (see Chapter 1).

have developed complex rules of inheritance and marriage systems, and these can often be understood in terms of the ecology of the particular society. For example, in many societies male reproductive success is linked to wealth and a father's inclusive fitness might be greater if a father concentrated his wealth in the hands of fewer of his male offspring rather than benefit them evenly. This is seen in some pastoralist societies where large herds of cattle are more viable than smaller ones and thus spreading cattle evenly might reproductively disadvantage all a man's sons. In such societies reproductive success is generally greater for older brothers than for younger ones. There are echoes of this approach seen in primogeniture (first-born son inherits all), which has been practised in some European societies. Parenthetically, the economic historian Gregory Clark believes that primogeniture helps to explain why the Industrial Revolution occurred initially in England: it created a population of well-educated but impoverished younger sons who sought status through trade and innovation.

Box 10.3   Genes and pair bonding

Some closely related species may have very different social structures. Humans and gibbons generally establish male–female pair bonds that last for considerable time and in essentially all human societies are the accepted cultural norm: chimpanzees have very different behaviours with no element of one to one male to female pair bonding.

These differences have been studied in voles and it has been shown that in a monogamous species, the prairie vole, vasopressin promotes and vasopressin antagonists inhibit pair-bond formation. The distribution of the vasopressin 1a receptor is very different in this monogamous species compared to that in the non-monogamous but closely related montane and meadow vole species. The coding sequence of the receptor is the same in all species of vole yet the 5′ regulatory sequence differs between the monogamous and non-monogamous species, suggesting different transcriptional regulation of the receptor. Molecular manipulation of this flanking sequence affects partner preference.

Polymorphisms in the 5′ flanking region of the human homologue, AVP receptor 1A, have been studied recently. There are associations between measures of male–female pair bonding and one particular repeat polymorphism (RS3). This association is restricted to males and is not found in females: similarly there were gender differences in the observations made in the voles with a greater effect present in the males. The RS3 allele was present in 40% of the population and was found to be associated with impaired pair bonding as reflected in marital problems, marital status, and spousal perception of the marriage. There was a greater effect if the individual male was homozygous for the allele but there was also an effect of heterozygosity, suggesting a dosage effect. Whereas an association study must always be interpreted with caution until it is repeated across populations, other studies have previously suggested that polymorphisms of the promoter region of the receptor are associated with an altered capacity for social interaction. They are also associated with different levels of activation of the amygdala, a component of the limbic system associated with pleasure and emotion.

Although the effect size is small, the study illustrates several points. First, fundamental components of human behaviour do have genetic determinants. Second, it is apparent that human behaviour has genetic and evolutionary relationships with analogous behaviours in other species. Third, evolution does lead to gender-specific behavioural effects. Fourth, the allele frequency of the polymorphism associated with impaired pair bonding is high at 40% and studies show that the alleles are distributed in accord with the Hardy–Weinberg equilibrium (see Chapter 2). This raises the intriguing possibility that humans evolved with two fitness-enhancing mating strategies and that an equilibrium exists between the two: one involving strong and enduring pair-bond formation, and one where pair-bond formation is less important, perhaps reflecting the mild polygny of past human society (see Chapter 7) and that male fitness can also be achieved and continues to be so through multiple serial or parallel relationships. In contrast, at least for this allele there appears to be no effect on the female strategy, which is optimized through sustained pair bonding.

Such studies, while at a very early stage, highlight the growing capacity that molecular genetics and evolutionary biology have to contribute to an understanding of the determinants of human behaviour.

10.4.5 Group behaviour and morality

Animals that live in groups have a set of behaviours that are necessary for harmony within the group. In some species, such as the hyena and wolf, this involves an obvious hierarchy within the group, with clear roles and rights for the alpha male or female. Humans live within a particularly intense group structure. This group structure evolved because it provided a fitness advantage for its individuals, probably for cooperative food gathering and defence against predators. Humpback whales hunt fish together in the phenomenon known as bubble net feeding, and fish school because it reduces the risk of any individual member being eaten.

Highly social species exhibit a number of behaviours that reinforce group bonds, such as grooming in the chimpanzee and sexual stimulation in the bonobo. Robin Dunbar and others have suggested that the evolution of language and gossip played a major role in generating and stabilizing bonds within early human groups. As group living requires multiple behaviours and is an integrated phenotype, all these selective pressures would have acted to determine the social and behavioural phenotype of our species. Natural selection, unlike artificial selection, is not acting on any one trait in isolation. Therefore, teasing apart and arguing for greater weight for one component or another is neither practical nor sensible.

But as we have already suggested, membership of a well-bonded social group requires that the rules of reciprocity are adhered to. Human groups are particularly sensitive to freeloaders or cheaters. We respond to cheating behaviour with exposure, ridicule, embarrassment, and punishment. Frameworks of what is acceptable and non-acceptable behaviour would become formalized within that group. As group size becomes greater than about 150, a formal internal structure is required for stability.

Concepts of morality are derived from these context-specific frameworks necessary to control freeloaders. They may be manifest in custom, taboos, rules, and tradition. But other factors also play an important role in a particular societal view of morality. These include rules and concepts imposed in part by hierarchical organizations to protect the hierarchy, and in part by formalization of belief systems.

10.4.6 Belief and religion

Every human society is characterized by a belief system that is reflected in its organization, tradition, and ritual. These belief systems generally involve some concept of the supernatural. Ritual burial implying a sense of afterlife has existed for at least 70 000 years.

Belief in the supernatural has been almost universal until modern rationalism emerged. The evolutionary question is whether belief in the supernatural has an adaptive advantage, or if it is simply the epiphenomenal outcome of other group behaviours. Supernatural belief is counter-factual and the adaptive advantage of suspending reality is not entirely clear. Its origin is also highly controversial. Perhaps it allowed individuals and the groups they were members of to develop an emotional stability in the face of events (such as drought) that they could not comprehend. Ritual, which often accompanies superstition, helps build group cohesion. Sagas and story-telling are often part of a belief system, and these may have helped reinforce group identify and thus cohesion. And belief in the supernatural as a potential source of punishment or reward could help a group deal with the problem of a freeloader.

The 30 000-year-old wall paintings in the caves of France and Spain may well be some of the earliest representations of ritual and belief. The organization of belief into formalized religion occurred in parallel with the development of larger population groups and the associated political organization. The issue of why and how belief in the supernatural arose has been the subject of considerable evolutionary reflection since the initial musings of Freud.

David Sloane Wilson and others have suggested that organized religion became a major way to control freeloaders and stabilize a large group. Some have argued that organized religion largely developed as a political tool within a hierarchical control system. Many societies have conflated, or even still do conflate, political rule and concepts of deity. Until the seventeenth century, British monarchs were considered to have divine powers of healing, and today they are still nominally head of an organized religious structure.

A common hypothesis is that religion evolved is a way of confronting the problem of inevitable death, and that complying with the group's behaviour would hopefully lead to a deferred reward. But Wilson also suggests that the religious group needs signs of commitment from the individual to comply in order to receive the rewards of group membership. This could take the form of sacrifices, tithes, or changed behaviour (for example, not eating meat on specific days). Paying a price to be a member of a group reduces the risk of being a freeloader. The risk of punishment for cheating is not only exclusion from the group but punishment by the supernatural. Wilson developed this hypothesis to argue that religion evolved through a group-selective process. This remains a controversial position. We have pointed out the adaptive value of reciprocal altruistic behaviour and group living for an individual. Within the context of the parallel processes of biological and cultural evolution, ritual and religion can be seen to have adaptive advantage for the individual and a group-selective argument is not necessary.

10.4.7 Learning

Humans are born in a relatively immature neurological state compared to other primates. Nevertheless, the human infant is not born with a total inability to perceive or react to its world, and is certainly not as immature as more altricial species such as the rat. A large amount of experimental and clinical data now show that human babies have very active sensory processes. They prefer symmetrical objects and images of an organized (rather than scrambled) face. Their sense of smell has also developed to the point that they can identify their mother. By the age of 9 months, babies are clearly able to recognize and respond to the psychological state of others, and by 15 months they can persuade a mother to react by pointing to an object.

Learning then becomes a process of acquiring skills and inducing changes during interactions with adults, which leads to new skills. Humans have evolved 'goal-based' imitative learning, which allows the growing child to learn about the goal and the actions necessary to reach that goal. Gradually this allows children to engage in their culture, and this process is greatly accelerated by the acquisition of language. By the age of 4 years children have moved to a level of cognitive development where at least a second level of intentionality can be demonstrated.

Learning from experience is a key adaptive capacity of many species, but is particularly well developed in humans. Learning by forming associations between events, called **associative learning**, is present even in adults and is a necessary precursor to inferential reasoning. The capacity to learn is regarded by some as simply another module of the mind in the context of orthodox evolutionary psychology (see section 10.5). Others regard it as flexible and generic, rather than domain-specific. Again, we see this as an unnecessary argument in the context of this book. Humans have evolved with a brain capable of assessing environmental information, storing information as memories and thus guiding decisions and consequent behaviour. Rather than trying to encode all possible responses in our genes, selection has endowed us with an advanced organic computer that can learn by association and experience, and make appropriate decisions. Indeed, in developmental learning, experience reinforces particular synaptic pathways and neuronal networks. Human learning is effectively a process of reinforcement by positive outcomes and avoidance following negative outcomes. Thus we learn to seek ripe fruits, but not to eat toadstools.

10.5 Evolutionary perspectives on psychology

We have highlighted how many aspects of human behaviour can be better understood by including evolutionary as well as cultural perspectives. But in doing so we have taken an integrated perspective: namely to what extent a behaviour can be considered to advance or protect fitness. The field of evolutionary psychology has also considered how the mind itself evolved. There are marked similarities in this discussion to considerations of how language evolved (see Chapter 6). Several schools of thought based in part on different approaches have emerged (see Box 10.4). Whereas the term evolutionary psychology can be used narrowly to describe a single one of these schools we will use it here in the broadest and most inclusive sense. Two extreme views exist: first, that the brain is a general tool able to flexibly respond to many situations, and alternatively that the brain has evolved as a series of domain-specific modules.

Box 10.4 The sociobiological debate and schools of evolutionary thought

In 1975, one of the most pre-eminent scholars of biology and evolutionary thought, E.O. Wilson, published a major book on animal behaviour entitled *Sociobiology: The New Synthesis*. The focus of the book was very much on animal behaviour, as Wilson was and is a particular expert on insect social behaviour and the issues of how cooperative behaviour developed in such species. But Wilson is a remarkable polymath and in the latter part of the book, where he was building on concepts such as kin selection, he discussed how evolutionary explanations and genetic determinants could explain a broad range of human behaviours. The debate that ensued became highly emotive and polarized. To argue for genetic determinism as the basis of human behaviour, irrespective of whether it had value when applied in other species, was seen as reinforcing arguments about race, and justifying eugenics, prejudice, and antisocial behaviours. It reinforced the perceived sterility of evolutionary thought.

Proponents of the genetic and the cultural positions became extremely polarized. A more balanced position emerged gradually, but there still remain a set of apparently distinct disciplines such as sociobiology, behavioural ecology, and evolutionary psychology, each with its own language and interpretations. Unfortunately, the side effect of all this is a range of terminologies that have made the field unnecessarily complex to the outsider. Much of this has been about territorial protection and reflects the different languages and theoretical bases of the different disciplines that have addressed the issue. The major schools of thought include the following.

- *Sociobiology* This applies evolutionary principles derived from studies in other species to an understanding of human nature. It relies on concepts such as kin selection, reciprocal altruism, and evolutionary game theory to interpret human behaviour.
- *Behavioural ecology* This uses the skill base of comparative ecology and ethology to question the basis of human behaviour. It seeks adaptive explanations for basic human behaviours.
- *Evolutionary psychology* This is based on the presumption that the human mind evolved during the Palaeolithic period in a context termed the environment of evolutionary adaptedness. It perceives the mind as a series of distinct evolved modules, and this has been the most dominant of the various approaches to understanding the human mind from an evolutionary perspective.

It should be apparent that, semantics and disciplinary pride aside, there is a strong overlap in each of these approaches. In this book, we have integrated these views where possible, or otherwise highlighted the debate. But clearly the human mind is an evolved structure, and its function has similarly evolved. How it functions is inherently the outcome of those evolved characteristics which include the very capacities which social scientists have focused upon: the capacity to learn and to respond to the social environment.

The most prominent advocates of the modular view are evolutionary psychologists Leda Cosmides and John Tooby. They proposed that there were strong selection pressures for each capacity of the mind to have evolved as independent modules. There were perhaps many thousands of modules, each for a different behaviour; for example, a module to detect freeloaders, a module to learn language, and so forth. A key concept in their thinking was that of the **environment of evolutionary adaptedness**. This was the putative environment that existed through the bulk of human existence, at least until the end of the Neolithic phase, during which selective pressures acted on human physiology and behaviour to lead to the current portfolio of human behaviours. The modular model implies that behaviours have an adaptive origin and must largely be genetically determined.

In contrast, the general model would suggest that most behaviours are learned, but can only be learned because of the evolved neural substrate. This dichotomy is an exaggeration made by advocates to make particular points and is to some extent unnecessary. What is clear is that humans have evolved with a neural infrastructure capable of learning, and with a series of cognitive abilities able to cope with novel situations and living within a complex social organization. But there is a stereotypy to a number of behaviours and emotions, and evidence for genetic determinants suggests that a finer grain of selection has operated. There is a renewed interest in the role of genetic assimilation (see Chapter 4) as a process by which learned behaviours are converted into genetically based behaviours. Indeed, the first description of what we now term genetic assimilation was named the Baldwin effect after the psychologist James Baldwin who was one of the first theorists to describe how behaviour might affect evolution.

Despite its limitations, the modular model does emphasize an important point. The human brain evolved under very different social and macro-environmental conditions to those in which humans now commonly live. If these modules were based on appropriate psychological adaptations when they evolved, then there will now be a mismatch between those modules and the modern constructed world. There would therefore be situations where the adaptations that underlie human behaviours have lost their adaptive advantage, and may

instead manifest as maladaptive pathologies. This argument has echoes of that used in Chapter 8 to describe the evolutionary origins of metabolic disease. Key to this school of thought has been the understanding of how the original selective circumstances led to a particular module of behaviour being selected. For example, a module for fear of dangerous animals such as snakes could be envisaged. Jealousy could also be conceived as a module that had an adaptive advantage, as a jealous individual was more likely to have a selective advantage over someone who took a passive view of being the victim of infidelity.

In the arguments over the origins of language, linguistic researchers view **universals** as having a selected origin and have therefore sought evidence for them across societies. Similarly there are obvious universals manifest in the human emotions, in the patterns of infant development, and in many aspects of social interactions such as mate choice and incest avoidance. These can be taken as evidence for an evolved mind. While there is considerable merit in this approach, the caveats we have expressed in Chapter 2 are equally valid here. Certainly, not all aspects of human biology need have an adaptive origin. There is a danger of falling into the trap of Just-So Stories, since spandrels and exaptations may apply equally to neural functions as they do to other aspects of biology. For example, while jealousy has been suggested to have an adaptive origin, there are no data to suggest it has a genetic underpinning and it might merely be the by-product of other brain capacities. Obviously there are limits to the empirical proof that is possible in evolutionary psychology (defined broadly), although this makes the science no less important.

It is important to note that the selective environments in which ancestral humans evolved were likely varied and changeable. There was no single environment of evolutionary adaptedness that acted as the selective bottleneck that led to the modern human mind. But nonetheless the concept does point out that some human behaviour may have had adaptive advantages in past times and may now be maladaptive. On the other hand, we must have a degree of psychological flexibility because if we were not adapted to the modern world we would have become extinct. In Chapter 6 we discussed the question of whether the human brain is still evolving.

10.6 Evolutionary psychiatry

Applying evolutionary principles to psychiatry builds on our previous discussion. Clearly, the various schools of evolutionary psychology are represented in how psychiatric states are potentially viewed. Because mental health disorders such as depression and anxiety are particularly common (perhaps affecting 25% of the Western population), it is necessary to consider why the evolved brain is vulnerable in the modern world. Some psychopathologies have a high frequency and cannot be explained by singular causes such as a monogenic trait. In these cases, their origin may be due to a discrepancy between the evolved biology and the actual environment, resulting in maladaptive consequences of a selected (adapted) trait. The key issue is the capacity to adapt to conditions requiring a particular behaviour. As with metabolic physiology, there are a range of psychological responses called upon to deal with a particular situation. Just as metabolic disease can develop when individuals live in environments with an energetic load beyond their selected capacity to cope (Chapter 8), psychological systems are limited in their capacity to adapt. These limitations may then be revealed in different societal or social conditions. The limits of this plasticity are genetically and thus evolutionarily determined. It is important to note that, irrespective of the conceptual model being used, specific genes do not link to specific behaviours, but rather to the functional neural networks that are involved. The debate between different schools of evolutionary psychology is essentially over the extent to which the brain remains plastic or is constrained in its plasticity by genetic determinants.

10.6.1 Personality traits and disorders

Personality can be defined as particular and somewhat inflexible ways of behaving. Individuals are recognized as having quite different personalities, and indeed we can recognize distinct personalities in domestic pets and in well-observed colonies of wild primates. One view of personality traits is that they represent constrained plasticity within the behavioural system. In general, evolutionary psychiatry presumes that a number of personality traits may have originated through adaptive advantage, but have become maladaptive in the current context. For example, a paranoid or anxious tendency may have

been helpful in avoiding predators. Risk-taking behaviour may have been advantageous in finding both a mate and new food supplies. When a personality trait is particularly exaggerated or constrained, it is considered pathological and is termed a **personality disorder**. Evidence from twin studies (despite their limitations) shows that even when reared apart, monozygotic twins exhibit concordance for a number of personality traits. This most probably reflects genetic determinants.

In evolutionary terms, individuals with **antisocial personality disorder** can be viewed as a manifestation of the cheater/freeloader. These individuals, whose personality often emerges in adolescence, are characterized by behaviours representing their willingness to take from the group without reciprocation. Game theory explains how cheaters can persist in a society made up primarily of reciprocators (see Box 10.2), and if they reproduce their genes will persist even if societies attempt to exclude them. A key feature of antisocial behaviour is the extent to which deception is used to hide it. It is inevitable that some cheaters will persist in any population.

It is important to distinguish this type of behaviour from **acting-out** behaviours of adolescence. As we have discussed in Chapter 7, such behaviours are transitional and arise because biological maturation precedes complete psychosocial maturation. Thus, adolescent acting-out behaviours occur during a period in the life cycle when there may be additional value in showing exploratory and risk-taking behaviour as a form of reproductive display. Indeed, males show a persistent tendency towards greater risk-taking behaviour throughout life. Many individuals can be seen as pushy and **attention-seeking**, or as impulsive or aggressive. Again, such behaviours could be seen to have had adaptive value in the mating game.

There are individuals who have difficulties in maintaining interpersonal relationships and have a poor self-image. As a result they may have a tendency towards suicidal or other self-damaging behaviours, inappropriate temper, and chronic feelings of emptiness. These individuals are unable to adapt to their social circumstance, often because they have a lack of insight, a limited capacity to interpret the circumstances they are in. This manifests as a pathology known as **borderline personality disorder**. Affected individuals are constrained in their ability to participate in their group and their behaviours can be perceived as unsuccessful attempts to be integrated and the unique juvenile period prior to sexual maturation. Human life is dependent on a complex web of interactions with other humans. We evolved with the capacity to interpret the actions of other members of our species, and to communicate and negotiate with them. The evolution of human behaviours can be understood in terms of the dynamics of mate choice, kin selection, reciprocal altruism, and social group living. Many human behaviours have evolved to address the challenge of a freeloader to the group.

Emotions are assumed to have evolved because they have had adaptive value for a social species, but they can become maladaptive with psychiatric consequences. This maladaptation may have arisen because of the massive change in the human social environment. Genetic or developmental variation may also impact on pathways determining behaviour. Either way, the match between the individual and the environment has changed.

KEY POINTS

- Human behaviour is built on selected and therefore genetically determined components of brain function.

- This evolved brain is the substrate on which individual experience and the current environment shape abilities and behaviour, giving humans the flexibility to exist in a wide range of societal environments.

- Humans are social animals characterized by living in groups larger than their immediate family. Selection has favoured traits which promoted fitness within this environment, such as cooperation, reciprocal altruism, and the abilities to interpret the actions of other members of our species and to detect freeloaders.

- Emotions have adaptive value for a social species, but they can become maladaptive with psychiatric consequences.

- Such maladaptations may have arisen because of changes in the human social environment, or because of genetic/developmental factors creating functional variation in pathways determining behaviour.

Further reading

Barkow, J.H., Cosmides, L., and Tooby, J. (1992) *The Adapted Mind: Evolutionary Psychology and the Generation of Culture*. Oxford University Press, New York.

Barrett, L., Dunbar, R., and Lycett, J. (2002) *Human Evolutionary Psychology*. Princeton University Press, Princeton, NJ.

Cartwright, J. (2000) *Evolution and Human Behaviour: Darwinian Perspectives on Human Nature*. Palgrave Press, London.

Hinde, R.A. (1999) *Why Gods Persist: a Scientific Approach to Religion*. Routledge, London.

Laland, K.N. and Brown, G.R. (2002) *Sense and Nonsense: Evolutionary Perspectives on Human Behaviour*. Oxford University Press, Oxford.

Marmot, M. (2004) *Status Syndrome: How Your Social Standing Directly Affects Your Health*. Bloomsbury Press, London.

Maynard Smith, J. (1982) *Evolution and the Theory of Games*. Cambridge University Press, Cambridge.

McGuire, M. and Troisi, A. (1998) *Darwinian Psychiatry*. Oxford University Press, Oxford.

Nesse, R.M. (2004) Natural selection and the pursuit of happiness. *Philosophical Transactions of the Royal Society of London Series B Biological Sciences* **359**, 1333–1347.

Sapolsky, R.M. (2001) *A Primates's Memoir*. Simon & Schuster, New York.

Sapolsky, R.M. (2005) The influence of social hierarchy on primate health. *Science* **308**, 648–652.

Weber, B.H. and Depew, D.J. (eds) (2003) *Evolution and Learning: The Baldwin Effect Reconsidered*. MIT Press, Cambridge, MA.

Wilkinson, R. and Marmot, M. (eds) (2003) *Social Determinants of Health: The Solid Facts*, 2nd edn. World Health Organization, Copenhagen.

Wilson, D.S. (2002) *Darwin's Cathedral: Evolution, Religion and the Nature of Society*. University of Chicago Press, Chicago, IL.

Wilson, E.O. (1975) *Sociobiology: The New Synthesis*. Belknap Press, Cambridge.